# The Anxiety and Stress Cure

Dr. Susan's Healthy Living
drsusanshealthyliving.com

Facebook.com/DrSusanRichards
drsusanshealthyliving@gmail.com
(650) 561-9978

Mention of specific companies or products in this book does not suggest endorsement by the author or publisher. Internet addresses and telephone numbers for resources provided in this book were accurate at the time it went to press.

ISBN 978-1511948913

Note: The information in this book is meant to complement the advice and guidance of your physician, not replace it. It is very important that any person who has medical problems be evaluated by a physician. If you are under the care of a physician, you should discuss any major changes in your regimen with him or her. Because this is a book and not a medical consultation, keep in mind that the information presented here may not apply in your particular case. In view of individual medical requirements, new research, and government regulations, it is the responsibility of the reader to validate health practices and treatments with a physician or health service.

# Acknowledgements

I want to give a huge thanks to my amazing editors Kendra Chun and Rebecca McLean for their incredibly helpful assistance with putting this book together. I also want to say thank you to Rebecca McLean for being my wonderful Art Director. I enjoyed working with both of them and found their help indispensable in creating this exceptional book.

# Table of Contents

Introduction .................................................................................................6

    A Self Help Approach to Anxiety and Stress Solutions .......................8

    How to Use This Book .....................................................................11

Part I:  Identifying the Problem .................................................................13

    Chapter 1: What Is Anxiety? ............................................................14

        The Emotions of Anxiety ..........................................................14

        The Common Causes of Anxiety ................................................15

        Types of Anxiety Disorders .......................................................15

        Risk Factors for Anxiety Disorders ...........................................22

        The Physiology of Anxiety ........................................................24

        Brain Chemistry ImbalancesThat May be Linked to Anxiety ......25

    Chapter 2: Physical Conditions That Can Cause Anxiety and Stress .......30

        Anxiety Due to Endocrine and Hormonal Imbalances ................30

        Anxiety Due to Immune System Imbalances ..............................40

        Anxiety Due to Cardiovascular System Disorders ......................43

Part II:  Evaluating Your Symptoms .........................................................45

    Chapter 3: The Anxiety and Stress Workbook .................................46

        Risk Factors for Anxiety ...........................................................49

        Key to Eating Habits ................................................................53

        Key to Exercise Habits .............................................................54

        Key to Major Life Stress Evaluation .........................................61

        Key to Daily Stress Evaluation .................................................64

    Chapter 4: Diagnosis of Anxiety and Panic Attacks .........................65

        Medical History .......................................................................66

        Physical Examination ...............................................................67

        Laboratory Testing ...................................................................67

Part III:  Finding the Solution ..................................................................73

    Chapter 5: My Diet for Relief of Anxiety and Stress .......................74

        Foods to Avoid .........................................................................75

        Foods That Help Relieve Anxiety ..............................................88

        Substitute Healthy Ingredients in Recipes ................................94

    Chapter 6: Menus, Meal Plans & Recipes ......................................103

        Breakfast Menus ....................................................................108

        Lunch and Dinner Menus .......................................................109

Breakfast Recipes ...................................................................111

Lunch and Dinner Recipes .....................................................122

Healthy Food Shopping List ...................................................140

Chapter 7: Vitamins, Minerals, Herbs & Essential Fatty Acids ...............142

Amino Acids for Relief of Anxiety...........................................144

Vitamins and Minerals for Relief of Anxiety...........................147

Herbal Relief for Conditions Related To Anxiety....................158

Essential Fatty Acids for Relief of Anxiety .............................169

Nutritional Supplements for Women with Anxiety and Stress ....................173

Chapter 8: Renewing Your Mind With Love, Peace and Joy ..................185

The Power of Prayer................................................................187

Love – The Great Healer..........................................................193

Embrace Gratitude and Appreciation .....................................197

Practice Forgiveness................................................................202

Live For Laughter ...................................................................205

Hold on to Happiness..............................................................228

The Gift of Giving...................................................................230

Chapter 9: Relaxation Techniques for Relief of Anxiety and Stress........218

How Stress Affects the Body ...................................................219

Techniques for Relaxation.......................................................219

Quieting the Mind and Body ..................................................220

Grounding Techniques ............................................................223

Releasing Muscle Tension .......................................................225

Erasing Stress and Tension .....................................................228

Healing the Inner Child ..........................................................230

Visualization ..........................................................................232

Affirmations ...........................................................................237

More Stress-Reduction Techniques for Anxiety ......................240

Putting Your Stress-Reduction Program Together...................241

Chapter 10: Breathing Exercises ...............................................................242

Putting Your Breathing Exercise Program Together................251

Chapter 11: Physical Exercises...................................................................252

The Benefits of Exercise ..........................................................252

Building Your Exercise Program .............................................260

Chapter 12: Stretches for Relief of Anxiety and Stress.............................266

Chapter 13: Acupressure for Relief of Anxiety and Stress .......................285

    About Acupressure .................................................................................285

    How to Perform Acupressure.................................................................286

Chapter 14: Treating Anxiety and Stress with Drugs .............................303

    Drugs as Appropriate Therapy ............................................................304

    Prescription Drugs .................................................................................307

    Drugs for PMS .......................................................................................314

    Drugs for Menopause ...........................................................................317

    Drugs for Hyperthyroidism.................................................................320

Chapter 15: How to Put Your Program Together.....................................324

    The Anxiety Workbook ........................................................................325

    Diet and Nutritional Supplements......................................................326

    Stress Reduction and Breathing Exercises .........................................326

    Physical Exercise....................................................................................327

    Conclusion..............................................................................................328

About Susan Richards, M.D............................................................................329

Notes.................................................................................................................330

Notes.................................................................................................................332

References .........................................................................................................333

# Introduction

**Dear Friend,**

I am thrilled that you have found my book, *The Anxiety and Stress Cure*, because I know that you are looking for positive and effective solutions to heal from these issues. I have written this book just for you, to share with you the all natural treatment program that I have developed for my own patients who were also suffering from the debilitating effects caused by anxiety, panic attacks and other stress related conditions.

My patients have come to me looking for solutions that would really work and would help restore emotional balance and elevate their mood. I have always loved working with my patients as a team effort and it has reaped great results! It has been very gratifying and heartwarming to see so many women regain their emotional and psychological health as well as eliminate the physical causes of anxiety symptoms. My patients have been thrilled with the terrific benefits that they received from following my program and I look forward to you receiving great benefits, too.

Emotional symptoms of anxiety, panic attacks and stress due to unhealed emotional issues, excessive life stresses and hormonal and chemical imbalances affect millions of people. While most of us experience anxiety, nervous tension, irritability, and edginess from time to time, it is often not a major interference in our lives. However, in extreme cases, the emotional and physical symptoms of anxiety and stress can be so severe that the people affected have a very difficult time functioning in their daily lives. In fact, almost 20 percent of the American population, 40 million people, suffer from anxiety symptoms each year.

The numbers are astonishing, especially since the symptoms of emotional distress are not limited to a particular age group. Rather, anxiety symptoms occur in people of all ages, from preadolescence to the postmenopausal years, but are twice as common in women as men. Thus, women have a greater susceptibility to the various emotional, chemical and hormonal imbalances that cause these symptoms.

When anxiety feelings are excessive, they can express themselves in episodes of fear, worry and panic. They may even trigger unpleasant physical symptoms such as rapid heartbeat, chest tightness, shortness of breath, digestive upset, and sleeplessness that can affect a person's ability to function well in the workplace, at home, and with co-workers, friends, and family. When experiencing an anxiety episode, it is difficult to organize and carry through with your activities. This can hamper effective performance in many different areas of life. You may also be struggling with some of these anxiety-related symptoms, too and are searching for relief.

## A Self-Care Approach to Relieving Anxiety and Stress

It has been a wonderful experience for me to have successfully treated many thousands of women patients who have come to me suffering from anxiety and other mood related symptoms. My patients have shared with me their fear, terror and, even frustration, when trying to deal with anxiety and panic attacks. They feel helpless, out of control and very concerned about these symptoms recurring and creating such havoc and upset in their lives. They will often try to avoid any situation that can trigger anxiety symptoms. This avoidance of anxiety can significantly limit their work, social life and even their range of personal relationships

Anxiety and stress symptoms stem from a broad range of emotional, social, chemical, and physical imbalances. Some people have anxiety episodes that are emotionally-based in childhood upsets and traumas, while others may develop stress symptoms after severe life crises such as a death, divorce, or job loss. Anxiety can also be a primary symptom of medical issues such as PMS, transition into menopause, hyperthyroidism, and hypoglycemia, as well as other health-related issues. Anxiety can also arise from nutritional deficiencies as well as substance use of drugs, alcohol, or overeating.

Women suffering from anxiety and panic attacks are usually treated in conventional medicine with drug therapies, sometimes combined with counseling or psychotherapy. Though anti-anxiety drugs help relieve the emotional symptoms, they can be a mixed blessing for many people. Often they produce unpleasant side effects as well as psychological and physical dependence. Counseling may be ineffective if underlying physical causes of anxiety are not adequately diagnosed. Many patients have told me of their fruitless search for adequate relief as they went from physician to physician, trying different combinations of medications.

Happily, I have found in working with thousands of women patients that anxiety, panic attacks and even phobias can be helped through alternative therapies. I have identified and eliminated dietary triggers of anxiety and developed therapeutic diets that help to balance mood and relieve anxiety. I have helped reduce my patients' stress response and supported a much healthier balance of their brain and body chemistry through the use of very effective nutritional supplements.

I have also shared with my patients a number of very effective and powerful anxiety and stress relieving techniques. These have included wonderful ways to transform and renew your mind through repatterning your thoughts, meditations, affirmations, visualization as well as anxiety relieving breathing exercises, stretches and pressure point therapy. I share all of these techniques that I have created and researched over the years with you in this book for you to benefit from.

Many of my patients have found that their lives were much more peaceful, calm and joyful as they followed my program and their anxiety symptoms began to diminish. For most patients, my self-care program gave them the relief that they were looking for. Some patients even found that they could reduce their dependence on mood altering medication or stop them altogether. Even in more severe cases of anxiety, the use of alternative therapies along with medication often produces far better results for patients than the use of medication alone. In addition, the practice of self-care techniques can greatly lessen the likelihood of the debilitating anxiety symptoms recurring. I have been delighted with the positive feedback that my patients have given me. They are always pleased and relieved to find that self-help treatments are so beneficial and effective.

## Lauren's Healing From Anxiety and Panic Attacks

I want to share with you one of my cases: my patient Lauren, a 33 year old woman, who was experiencing such severe anxiety and panic attacks that they drastically affected the quality of her life. Her social anxiety was so severe that she had curtailed her social life and was finding excuses to avoid seeing friends. She dreaded visits with her family who she found to be overbearing and domineering. She worried endlessly about spending time with her mother and father for family holidays because she felt that they disapproved of her career as a graphic artist.

Lauren also suffered from shortness of breath, chest pain, frequent urination, headaches and insomnia when her symptoms were at their worst. She tried counseling and talk therapy but didn't have much success in relieving her symptoms. She came to me seeking relief from her symptoms through natural therapies, hoping to avoid medication, if at all possible. Upon taking a patient history, I found that Lauren also suffered from moderately severe PMS (premenstrual syndrome) symptoms for a week and a half each month including uncomfortable anxiety, mood swings, irritability, bloating, and sugar cravings during this time. She was also eating a diet that was worsening her anxiety symptoms including lots of sugary desserts and snacks, including hot chocolate in the evening and coffee.

I created a therapeutic program for Lauren that provided her with the dietary and nutritional support that she needed to help relieve her anxiety and stress symptoms, eliminate her symptoms of PMS and promote a more balanced brain and hormonal chemistry. She also started to practice the positive mind repatterning therapies, meditations and breathing techniques that I shared with her as well as beginning a daily walking program.

Lauren found that she loved doing the repatterning techniques and felt that they were making a real difference in how she handled situations that would normally trigger anxiety. She also joined a support group that she found very beneficial. Attending this group started to help relieve her social anxiety. Lauren felt as she continued on with the program that she was becoming more positive and optimistic and was becoming less burdened by fear and worry. She began to feel more peaceful and calm and became more confident in her ability to manage stress. Her relationship with her parents also improved. Lauren found that she was able to share her feelings and concerns with them without fear of their disapproval. I was thrilled by all of the positive steps that she was making in her life as her anxiety symptoms began to diminish.

Like Lauren, the end result of my program can also help to provide you with relief from your anxiety symptoms and promote much improved physical health, too, whether you choose to work with your doctor and take antianxiety medications or only want to work with these beneficial natural therapies. Either treatment pathway can provide you with excellent results, depending on what will be most effective for you. I discuss both my all natural program as well as the medical therapies for anxiety, panic attacks and stress symptoms in great detail in this book.

## How to Use This Book

I feel strongly that any woman interested in healing from anxiety, panic attacks and other stress symptoms should have access to this information. Because there are many women whom I will never see as patients in my medical practice, I wrote this book to share the program that I have developed and found, through years of medical practice, to be most useful. I hope you will find this information as useful as my patients have. I am continuously expanding my own knowledge about the most up-to-date therapies and researching new healthcare techniques for treating these issues.

My program includes my anxiety relief diet as well as the vitamins, minerals, essential fatty acids, amino acids and herbs that I have found to be the most effective in eliminating my patient's symptoms and restoring a healthy brain, nervous system and hormonal balance. Following a therapeutic dietary and nutritional supplement program is very beneficial for successfully relieving anxiety and stress and promoting a relaxed, calm and joyful mood. It will be very helpful in assisting you to successfully navigate the day-to-day stresses of your life.

I also share with you wonderful techniques to help reduce anxiety through positive repatterning of your emotions and feelings as well as meditations, affirmations, visualizations and deep breathing exercises that promote peace, relaxation and joy. I have included acupressure massage points, stretching exercises and recommendations for physical exercise that are specifically helpful for the relief of anxiety and stress. The book also contains important chapters on the symptoms, risk factors and medical diagnosis of these issues. I also discuss the most up to date drug therapies for anxiety, panic attacks and stress symptoms and explain the pros and cons of all the medical treatments.

I recommend that you read through the entire book first to familiarize yourself with the material. The Anxiety Workbook (Chapter 3) will help you evaluate your symptoms, risk factors, and stress-creating lifestyle habits. Next, turn to the therapy chapters and read through the rest of the book. Try all the therapies that most appeal to you and pertain to your symptoms. Establish a regimen that works for you and follow it every day.

My anxiety and stress healing program is practical and easy to follow. You may use it by itself or in conjunction with a medical program. While working with a physician or psychologist may be necessary to establish a definitive diagnosis of the causes of anxiety, and medical therapy may still be necessary if you have more severe symptoms, my treatment program will help to correct and balance the chemical and hormonal imbalances that trigger these issues in the first place. This book will not only help speed up the diagnostic process but also bring you significant relief.

My treatment program can play a major role in reducing your anxiety symptoms and preventing their recurrence. The feelings of peace and wellness that can be yours with this self-care program will radiate out and touch your whole life. I hope that your life is positively transformed by these beneficial therapies.

Love,

Dr. Susan

# Part I:
# Identifying the Problem

# 1

## What Is Anxiety?

I want to begin our journey together of supporting your healing from anxiety and stress by giving you important information about these conditions. In this chapter, I describe the symptoms of anxiety, panic attacks and other stress-related issues. I also discuss the risk factors that can predispose you towards developing these conditions. This will help you to better understand your stress-related symptoms and what might be triggering them. I also discuss the chemical and physiological imbalances that can occur with anxiety and stress.

The word anxiety means "a state of being worried, uneasy or apprehensive about what may happen." It is also described as a "feeling of being powerless and unable to cope with threatening events . . . [characterized] by physical tension." Though this is a dictionary definition, it certainly fits the way that many women feel about their lives today. The frequency with which women feel anxiety is reflected in my medical practice: My patients complain about anxiety and other emotional symptoms more than anything else. This is true whether they are seeking help for primarily psychological or physical ailments.

### The Emotions of Anxiety

Anxiety for most of us is an inevitable part of life. We all encounter every day, real life situations to which anxiety is a reasonable response. These situations can be as major as a death, divorce, or job loss, or as seemingly minor as going to the doctor or meeting new people at a social event. Although anxiety is a very common emotional response, its expression can take different forms. It varies in intensity from being an appropriate response to stressful or difficult situations to being an actual psychiatric disorder. Disorders can occur when symptoms persist or are severe in nature. Some women have anxiety symptoms so intense that the symptoms interfere with their ability to function on a day-to-day basis.

## The Common Causes of Anxiety

When a woman identifies anxiety as a serious complaint, any of four body systems may be compromised:

- *The brain and nervous system*, which includes the emotional centers of the brain and the fibers that connect the brain, organs, and muscles by transmitting impulses that allow normal bodily sensation and movement, as well as the experience and expression of moods and feelings.

- *The endocrine or glandular system*, which regulates reproductive and metabolic functions, such as menstruation and the efficient burning of food for energy. The endocrine glands communicate with one another by secreting into the bloodstream chemicals called hormones that carry chemical messages from one gland to another.

- *The immune system*, which fights foreign invaders in the body, such as bacteria, viruses, and cancer cells.

- *The cardiovascular system*, which consists of the heart and all the blood vessels in the body.

The remainder of this chapter and the following chapter discuss the most common psychological and physical problems in these systems that I have encountered over the years in my medical practice that can cause anxiety symptoms. Many (but not all) of them are problems often seen by any physician practicing primary care medicine. Most likely your symptoms of anxiety are related to one or more of these health problems.

## Types of Anxiety Disorders

Three major types of psychologically based anxiety disorders are very pertinent to women: generalized anxiety disorder, panic disorder, and phobias. Research in brain chemistry has shown that these anxiety disorders may also be linked to specific chemical changes in the brain, thus suggesting a strong mind-body link. The field of psychiatry also recognizes other types of anxiety disorders, such as obsessive-compulsive disorder and post-traumatic stress syndrome. While there tends to be some overlap in the symptoms experienced by women with the various types of anxiety disorders, there are still significant differences among the specific types. Let's now look at the different types of anxiety-related conditions.

## *Generalized Anxiety Disorder*

Generalized anxiety disorder is characterized by chronic anxiety that tends to focus on real life issues, such as problems with work, finances, relationships, or health, which feel dangerous or threatening to a woman's security and well-being. The emotional and physical symptoms of anxiety that these situations elicit must persist for at least six months to establish this diagnosis. Often, the real life issues in turn elicit deeper emotional concerns, such as fear of abandonment, rejection, or not being loved. These deep fears may underlie the anxiety around troubled personal relationships, fear of failure, inability to cope effectively with stressful situations, and even fear of death when there are health concerns. Since the symptoms are experienced frequently, they can interfere with a woman's quality of life and her ability to function optimally on a daily basis.

Common symptoms include frequent upset, worry, and nervous tension, as well as insomnia, irritability, difficulty concentrating, and startling easily. Physical symptoms include the typical fight-or-flight response of rapid heartbeat, cold hands and feet, shortness of breath, muscle tension, shakiness, depression, and chronic fatigue. The symptoms, however, are not so severe as to be complicated by panic attacks and phobias. Generalized anxiety disorder can date back as early as childhood, but a majority of patients are initially diagnosed in their twenties or thirties. The disorder seems to occur with equal frequency among both men and women.

Consult a physician if you suffer from an apparent generalized anxiety disorder to rule out any possible medical disorders that could be causing these symptoms. For example, hyperthyroidism, food allergies, or PMS are often mistaken for an anxiety disorder. In addition, since anxiety and depression can coexist, it is important to know which is the primary component, as treatment can differ depending on which is primary and which is secondary.

## *Panic Disorder*

The experience of panic is characterized by the sudden onset of intense fear or apprehension that occurs unexpectedly for no apparent reason. Usually the panic symptoms appear without prior warning, catching a person unaware; a woman is often in the middle of a panic episode before she even has time to register what is happening. Luckily, the acute phase of the panic attack tends to be short-lived, lasting only a few minutes. However, the symptoms may persist beyond the initial attack, though at a level of lesser intensity.

To have the diagnosis of panic disorder, a woman must have experienced at least four panic attacks in a one-month period, or have experienced significant apprehension and worry throughout an entire month following a single panic attack. As in generalized anxiety disorder, the symptoms are typical of the fight-or-flight reaction, although panic attacks tend to be much more intense and disabling.

Since panic attacks are acute and short-lived, they also differ in duration from generalized anxiety disorder, where the symptoms are persistent and chronic. Typical symptoms include at least four of the following: rapid heartbeat or heart palpitations, chest pain, shakiness, dizziness, faintness, shortness of breath, cold hands and feet, numbness and tingling in the hands and feet, intestinal distress, sweating, feelings of losing control, and feelings of unreality.

Between panic episodes, women can suffer much fear and apprehension, worrying about their recurrence. Panic disorder tends to coexist with agoraphobia (fear of open spaces or public places), which is also discussed in this chapter. In fact, panic attacks in combination with agoraphobia affect 5 percent of the population in this country, while only 1 percent suffers from panic disorder alone. Panic disorder tends to develop during the twenties in susceptible women.

It is important to differentiate panic disorder from medical problems such as mitral valve prolapse (which can coexist with panic disorder and produce similar symptoms) and hypoglycemia, or even chemical imbalances like drug withdrawal or excessive caffeine intake. A careful diagnostic evaluation should be done by a physician to make sure that a medical problem has not been overlooked or misdiagnosed.

## Phobias

Phobias are characterized by an excessive, persistent, and often irrational fear of a person, object, place, or situation. In severe cases, the person suffering from a particular phobia will try to avoid the inciting trigger. At the very least, a phobia can create severe emotional distress and can cause a person to postpone facing situations that trigger the phobia. Day-to-day functioning or even one's health and well-being can be compromised, particularly when the phobia centers on being in public places, going to social gatherings, giving public speeches, or even seeing a doctor or dentist.

As mentioned earlier, agoraphobia (fear of open or public spaces) is fairly prevalent in our society, affecting 5 percent of the population to some degree. In fact, it is the most common of all the anxiety disorders. Approximately three-quarters of all agoraphobics are women. Women with agoraphobia may develop a panic attack when placed in such common situations as using public transportation (buses, airplanes, trains), being in public places like department stores, shopping malls, and crowded restaurants, or being in confined spaces such as tunnels. In all these cases, an overriding concern is the fear of being trapped in a place where escape is difficult and being overcome by a panic attack. Many women are also concerned about the reactions people around them may have if a panic attack occurs.

As the phobia becomes worse, even thinking about being in a situation to which one has a phobic reaction can engender panic. As a result, women with agoraphobia often begin to restrict their range of activities and locations. In extreme cases, they may only venture out when accompanied by a trusted friend or relative. Some agoraphobics are even afraid to be alone in their own homes unless a companion remains with them. Luckily, agoraphobia is an easily treated condition if the appropriate therapy is undertaken. A combination of medication, stress management training and counseling will produce good results in as many as 90 percent of all people suffering from this condition.

Another common type of phobia is social phobia. This occurs when there is fear of performing in front of other people or being scrutinized by other people. The most common social phobia involves public speaking. This is a major issue for many people, including students giving speeches in class, women who must give a formal presentation at work or at social or charitable functions, and even professional actors and other performers.

Other common social phobias include fear of eating in public, fear of being watched or looked at while at social gatherings, fear of signing documents in front of other people, fear of being photographed in a crowded room, or even fear of blushing in public. These phobias may begin in childhood and can persist throughout adult life (although in many women, social phobias decrease in severity with age). They often develop in children who are more shy and self-conscious.

Many people engage in a variety of self-help techniques to deal with social phobias, some of which are remarkably effective. For example, amateur and professional speaking groups and organizations give people the chance to speak in front of a supportive peer group; this often helps decrease anxiety related to public speaking. Classes on self-image and self-esteem utilize a variety of imaging and assertiveness techniques; these classes tend to be very popular and well-attended. Some women find that they can effectively dispel social phobias when engaged in one-on-one counseling.

A third type of phobia, called simple phobia, involves fear of a particular situation or object. Common examples of simple phobias include fear of animals like dogs or snakes, airplanes (for fear the airplane will crash), heights, or even having blood drawn for a medical test. Many simple phobias originate in childhood and persist into adult life (even though the adult may recognize that they are irrational). They may also originate in a traumatic event, such as being stuck in an elevator or experiencing a near accident during plane travel. A traumatic event may condition a person to fear repeated exposure to a similar situation (e.g., plane travel or using an elevator).

Simple phobias are easiest to treat, because the fear response can usually be handled by gradual exposure to the phobia-inducing situation or object as well as the practice of a variety of stress-reducing techniques such as visualizations and affirmations. These are discussed in the self-help section of this book.

### Obsessive-Compulsive Disorder

Obsessive-compulsive disorder (OCD) is a condition characterized by unwanted irrational thoughts and fears (obsessions) that cause you to do repetitive behavior (compulsions). Examples of the types of irrational thoughts often seen with OCD can include mundane repeated worries about whether you've locked the door before leaving the house or turned off the stove to avoid starting a fire in the house to extreme irrational fears about bodily harm or even death.

Other disorders linked to this condition include an obsession with how one looks with the belief of being ugly or having an abnormally shaped body part such as excessive worrying about the size and shape of one's breasts. With hypochondria, a woman may worry repeatedly about developing a serious illness , even if there is no realistic foundation for this belief. The compulsive behavior can involve checking over and over again to make sure that the tasks like locking the door or turning off the stove have been carried out. Other common compulsive behavior can include repeated calls to loved ones to make sure that they are safe or fear of germs; which leads people with this issue to constantly wash their hands for fear of catching an infection.

Women with OCD may realize that their obsessions aren't reasonable and may even try to ignore them, but this only increases their feelings of anxiety and stress that this condition causes. As a result, women will commonly give in to their concerns and engage in compulsive behavior to try to ease their feelings of anxiety and even panic. This leads to more of the ritualistic behavior that is typical of this condition.

## Post-Traumatic Stress Disorder

Post-traumatic stress disorder (PTSD) is a severe anxiety condition that can develop after a person is exposed to one or more traumatic events, such as a serious injury, sexual assault, car accident, domestic abuse, war or, in extreme cases, the threat of death. Women are more likely than men to develop PTSD in response to a traumatic incident.

One woman may experience a very stressful event and still recover and never develop PTSD while another woman who experiences the same situation may have a heightened stress reaction that doesn't heal or diminish with time, leaving her emotionally ravaged with recurring symptoms. To have the diagnosis of PTSD, the following symptoms much last for at least three months or more without relief unless effective treatment is instituted.

Women with PTSD suffer from three types of disturbing symptoms. These include recurring flashbacks in which you may constantly relive the event, disturbing your day-to-day activities. You may also have repeated nightmares of the traumatic event or strong reactions to situations that remind you of the event.

A second type of reaction is avoidance in which there is emotional numbing or detachment from the event. If you have this type of response, you may not be able to remember important parts of the event. You may tend to avoid people, places or thoughts that remind you of the trauma. This can continue for more than a month after the traumatic event has occurred.

In contrast, if you develop hypervigilance, you may always be scanning your environment for imminent sign of danger. You probably tend to startle easily and may even have difficulty concentrating. Difficulty falling or staying asleep is very common as are other symptoms of anxiety and stress.

## Risk Factors for Anxiety Disorders

A variety of factors can predispose a woman to develop anxiety disorders. These include major long- and short-term life stresses, genetic factors (familial predisposition), family programming, and personal belief systems as well as physiological and chemical imbalances within the brain and nervous system.

### Genetic Factors (Familial Predisposition)

Genetic factors seem to have some relevance as risk factors for developing anxiety disorders. For example, in studies of identical twins, the likelihood of both twins having an anxiety disorder if one is afflicted is statistically significant (greater than 30 percent). Fraternal twins, who do not have the same genetic makeup, are also at higher risk of developing an anxiety disorder if their sibling is affected, although they do not have nearly the risk of identical twins. Agoraphobia, the most common anxiety disorder, also seems to show a familial predisposition. While 5 percent of the entire population suffers from this condition, the rate of agoraphobia in people with one parent who had this diagnosis is 15 to 25 percent.

### Family Programming

Certain types of family environments seem to predispose children to develop anxiety disorders, producing insecurity, fear, and dependency in susceptible children. One such setting is created by parents who are critical perfectionists, constantly demanding that a child perform at peak levels. In this family, any departure from peak performance is punished or criticized. A child in this situation may grow up with a poor sense of self-esteem, anxious and afraid to take risks for fear of failing.

Parents who themselves have phobias or are overly anxious may also raise children who suffer from anxiety. These parents tend to teach their children that the world is a fearful place, full of danger and risks. This type of family may raise a child who is timid and anxious about meeting new life challenges.

Parents who are overly controlling and suppress a child's self-assertiveness by punishment may engender anxiety in their children. Such children may grow up afraid to take initiative or show their true convictions. In this environment, children are punished for speaking out and expressing their feelings. Not all children raised in stressful family environments develop anxiety disorders. Many children grow up in very difficult family environments without ever suffering excessive anxiety. The likelihood of developing an anxiety disorder when raised in a high-stress family is probably greater in children born with more sensitive and reactive personalities. These are children whose fight-or-flight response is easily triggered by upsetting circumstances.

## Major Life Stresses

Women who have suffered from major life stresses over a long period of time, such as marriage to an abusive husband, death, chronic illness in several family members, or constant financial worries, may find their ability to handle stress with equanimity and calm hampered. Unremitting major life stresses are likely to cause wear and tear on the nervous system and, over time, cause a woman to be excessively anxious or tense.

In addition, a major stress occurring in a short period of time can also produce anxiety. This is particularly true when the stressor—such as death of a spouse or loss of a long-term job—causes significant life change or dislocation. Even positive experiences such as getting married or having a baby can cause anxiety, because they throw people into entirely new situations for which they may have no preparation.

## Personal Belief Systems

Many women have belief systems that reinforce the anxiety disorders and engender behavior that maintains the anxiety state. These include poor self-image and a low estimate of one's abilities. Many women with anxiety disorders are very insecure and feel ill-equipped to make the life changes necessary to confront and change anxiety-related issues.

Women with anxiety disorders often hold a negative view of the world. They see life situations and places as dangerous and threatening, whereas women without anxiety disorders may see the same circumstances as harmless and benign. These negative belief systems about the outside world, if too ingrained, may make it difficult to change.

In addition, women with anxiety disorders often reinforce their own upset through their internal dialogue. A woman who engages in constant fearful and anxious self-talk may anticipate certain situations and people as threatening and dangerous, thus reinforcing her feelings of anxiety. Because we are all constantly dialoguing with ourselves throughout much of the day, negative self-talk can be a big factor in perpetuating anxiety disorders.

## The Physiology of Anxiety

While most women experience anxiety emotionally as upset and distress, we also react to these upsetting feelings on a physical level. What actually happens to our body when we are feeling anxious, nervous, or even panicky? Anxiety feelings normally set off an alarm reaction in our body called the "fight-or-flight" response. This response occurs to any perceived threat, whether it is physically real, psychologically upsetting, or even imaginary. Our thoughts and feelings can trigger this response; it can even occur simply when we're excited. The fight-or-flight response is a powerful, protective mechanism that allows your body to mobilize energy quickly and escape from or confront any type of danger.

The fight-or-flight response begins in our nervous system. The nervous system consists of the brain, the spinal cord, and the peripheral nerves. It is divided by function into two parts: the voluntary nervous system and the involuntary (or autonomic) nervous system.

The voluntary nervous system manages activity in the conscious domain. For example, if you place your hand on a hot stove, pain fibers will trigger a response that is sent to the brain. The brain sends back an immediate response telling you to move your hand before you burn yourself. You then pull your hand away, fast.

The autonomic nervous system regulates functions of which the average person is usually unaware, such as muscle tension, pulse rate, respiration, glandular function, and the circulation of the blood. The autonomic nervous system is also divided into two parts that oppose and complement each other: the sympathetic and parasympathetic nervous systems. These control the upper and lower limits of your physiology, respectively. For example, if excitement speeds up the heart rate too much, the parasympathetic nervous system's job is to act as a control circuit and slow it down. If the heart slows down too much, then the sympathetic nervous system's job is to speed it up.

A fight-or-flight response stimulates the sympathetic nervous system, triggering several different physical responses. Our adrenal glands increase their output of adrenaline and cortisone as body chemistry adjusts to meet the crisis. The outpouring of these hormones causes the heart and pulse rate to speed up, the breathing to become shallow and rapid, and the hands and feet to become icy cold. In addition, muscles tighten up and become tense and contracted. The sympathetic nervous system also triggers the release of stored sugar in the liver, an increase in the metabolic rate of the body, inhibition of digestion, and an excess secretion of acid in the stomach—all in response to feelings of anxiety and stress.

Though the physiological response to anxiety or stress is the same no matter what the initial stressor is (physical danger, psychological distress, or imaginary threat), the chemical trigger for anxiety can vary greatly. For example, the chemical imbalance that triggers PMS-related anxiety is often quite different from the chemical or hormonal imbalances seen in hyperthyroidism or menopause-related anxiety. I will discuss the chemical triggers as I explore the common causes of anxiety.

In women with anxiety or panic episodes, the sympathetic nervous system is actually too sensitive or too easily triggered. Their systems are too often in a state of readiness to react to a crisis. This puts them in a constant state of tension, fight-or-flight.

## Brain Chemistry Imbalances That May be Linked to Anxiety

While no one brain chemical imbalance has been found to be a definitive cause of anxiety and stress, much is now known about the chemistry of the brain and how the complex interplay between these chemicals can significantly affect our mood and emotions. Within the brain, we produce chemicals that calm us down and relax us as well as chemicals that can cause a state of arousal, energy and zest for life.

When these substances are produced in healthy balance, we can experience a wide range of emotions that feel positive and life affirming. However, if these chemicals are out of balance in either direction, it can lead to panic and anxiety on one end and depression, low mental energy and sadness on the other. Let's look at the chemical imbalances that may be linked to anxiety, panic attacks and other stress related conditions.

Serotonin and dopamine are neurotransmitters, chemicals that are naturally occurring and relay electrical messages between nerve cells throughout your body. Serotonin is part of the inhibitory pathway, while dopamine is part of the excitatory pathway. Because these two pathways oppose and complement one another, imbalances in either serotonin or dopamine can make a person more sensitive to everyday stress than someone who is able to produce these neurochemicals in more balanced and appropriate amounts.

**Serotonin** is one of your brain's principal neurotransmitters. Its action on the nerves is inhibitory, relieving stress and calming the mind. Serotonin also regulates appetite, influences mood, and promotes healthy hormone production.

**Dopamine** is a neurotransmitter that stimulates and energizes the body. In fact, dopamine is actually a precursor to substances made by the adrenal medulla and sympathetic nervous system that regulate the stress response within the body. High levels of dopamine have been linked to such traits as mental alertness, physical energy, and vitality, as well as aggressive drive and libido. Dopamine is synthesized by the adrenal glands and is converted by the body into the stress hormones epinephrine and norepinephrine, which also stimulate hormone production. Before ages 40 to 45, dopamine levels remain fairly stable, but they then decrease by about 13 percent per decade.

As levels of these neurotransmitters begin to decline with age, your body's ability to handle stressful events can change. Depressed serotonin levels can trigger mood imbalances, sleeplessness, and food cravings. For example, women who suffer from PMS may have a tendency towards low serotonin levels. That's one reason why women with PMS often respond to stressful events in an exaggerated manner. Irritability, anger, tension, and upset are common responses in the second half of the menstrual cycle to such usually small stresses as a nagging child, a minor disagreement with a spouse, or a work deadline. Women who suffer from a serotonin imbalance often feel like a firecracker about to explode for one to two weeks out of each month.

Similarly, panic disorders have been identified as occurring in animals when there is a dysfunction in a specific system in the brain called the noradrenergic system. This system is very sensitive to an excitatory neurotransmitter called norepinephrine. Like dopamine, norepinephrine triggers arousal and overactivity within the brain and nervous system. When there is a dysfunction in the way the noradrenergic system functions, panic attacks are triggered.

In contrast, when levels of the stimulatory neurotransmitter dopamine are depressed, epinephrine and norepinephrine production is also diminished. This is more common in women who are frequently depressed, fatigued, lethargic, and lack vital force and joy of life.

**GABA**. Research suggests that women with generalized anxiety disorder may have an imbalance of gamma amino butyric acid (GABA) in their brain. GABA is an inhibitory neurotransmitter, a substance that transmits messages from one part of the brain to another. GABA acts as a chemical brake within the brain, helping to shut down overactivity, typically seen with anxiety and panic attacks.

When people are given GABA or placed on drugs that increase the activity of GABA; their anxiety is diminished. While the exact mechanism triggering generalized anxiety is not known, it is possible that a GABA deficiency or extreme sensitivity on the part of the body to the available GABA levels may play a role in its etiology.

**Taurine**. This amino acid helps to promote feelings of peace and calm and prevents the overactivity that can occur when the excitatory neurotransmitters are out of balance. Taurine helps to support restful sleep and is useful in the control of anxiety and bipolar disorder. It also helps to control seizure disorders. Its activity is similar to that of the inhibitory neurotransmitter, GABA. Women may be more prone towards anxiety and panic attacks if taurine levels are low.

Taurine is produced within the body from two other amino acids and can also be obtained from foods such as meat and fish. Animal research studies have shown significant antianxiety benefits of taurine. In one study, animals treated with taurine spent more time in open areas and less time backing away from anxiety-provoking situations.

Taurine also helps to move important minerals like potassium, calcium and magnesium in and out of the heart, thereby enhancing heart health. As a sulfur containing amino acid, it is necessary for the process of detoxification. Taurine conjugates or binds with bile acids to maintain the solubility of fats and cholesterol in bile, thereby helping to prevent the formation of gallstones.

**Melatonin**. This is a hormone produced from serotonin and secreted by the pineal gland. Its secretion takes place at night and is inhibited by light. As such, it sets and regulates the timing of your body's natural circadian rhythms, such as waking and sleeping. Unfortunately, as you get older, you produce less and less melatonin. This is due, in part, to menopause.

Women who have poor sleep patterns, such as night shift workers, are also more likely to have decreased melatonin production. Finally, women who suffer from anxiety, panic attacks and phobias may also have sleep disturbances and insomnia due to melatonin imbalances. I have seen women as young as their twenties and thirties benefit from melatonin supplementation, if they were prone to anxiety and panic episodes.

For melatonin to be effective, your bedroom should be dark, as light suppresses its release. Drugs such as aspirin, ibuprofen, beta-blockers, calcium channel blocks, sleeping pills and tranquilizer may deplete melatonin levels.

**Noradrenergic system**. Panic disorders have been identified as occurring in animals when there is a dysfunction in a specific system in the brain called the noradrenergic system. This system is very sensitive to an excitatory neurotransmitter called norepinephrine. Like dopamine, norepinephrine triggers arousal and overactivity within the brain and nervous system (as does another excitatory chemical called epinephrine). When there is a dysfunction in the way the noradrenergic system functions, panic attacks are triggered. This is also thought to be a cause of anxiety and stress reactions in humans, as well.

In contrast, when levels of the stimulatory neurotransmitter dopamine are depressed, epinephrine and norepinephrine production is also diminished. This is probably more common in women who are frequently depressed, fatigued, lethargic, and lack vital force and joy of life.

In summary, anxiety disorders can take a variety of forms, including generalized anxiety disorder, panic disorder, and phobias. Many circumstances can increase the risk of developing an anxiety disorder, such as physiological imbalances, genetic factors, family upbringing, major long- and short-term life stress, and the person's own personal beliefs and negative self-talk, which can keep an anxiety disorder going once it has become an established process. Fortunately, anxiety disorders can be treated through counseling, stress management techniques and breathing exercises, nutritional therapies, and regular exercise. These are discussed in depth in the self-help chapters of this book.

In the next chapter, we will look at physical conditions that are also frequently linked to anxiety and stress reactions.

# 2

## Physical Conditions That Can Cause Anxiety and Stress

In this chapter, I discuss a number of physical conditions that can commonly cause symptoms of anxiety, panic attacks and stress. It is very important for you to be aware of these conditions. Not only can they co-exist with emotional causes of anxiety but sometimes they can be the main cause of your symptoms.

The physical causes of anxiety must be properly diagnosed by your doctor or caregiver so that you receive the correct treatment. Otherwise you may be diagnosed as having an emotional anxiety disorder while the true cause of your symptoms isn't identified. This can cause severe health problems. Once these physical causes of anxiety are treated, the symptoms due to these conditions may be totally eliminated. These include endocrine, hormonal and metabolic disorders, immune system imbalances and cardiovascular system disorders.

### Anxiety Due to Endocrine and Hormonal Imbalances

Many endocrine-related health problems have anxiety and mood swings as major symptoms. These health conditions are discussed in this section.

*Premenstrual Syndrome*

Anxiety and mood swings are the hallmark of premenstrual syndrome (PMS), one of the most common problems affecting women during their reproductive years (from the teens to the early fifties). In fact, it affects one-third to one-half of American women in this age group. In my practice, more than 90 percent of women with PMS complain of heightened anxiety and irritability that increases in intensity varying from several days to the week or two prior to menstruation.

Many PMS patients describe mood and personality changes that occur during this time. Even if they are normally calm and patient, they may become irritable and more moody as their menstrual period approaches. My patients have told me that they are impatient and irritable with their children, pick fights with their spouses, and snap at friends and co-workers. Some spend the rest of the month repairing the emotional damage done to their relationships during this time.

In addition to the emotional symptoms, PMS has numerous physical symptoms involving almost every system in the body. More than 150 symptoms have been documented, including headaches, bloating, breast tenderness, weight gain, sugar craving, and acne. However, for many women, the emotional symptoms and fatigue are the most severe, adversely affecting their family relationships and their ability to work. In addition, it is not unusual for women to have as many as 10 to 12 of the symptoms.

There is no single hormonal or chemical imbalance has been linked to PMS. Instead, over two dozen hormonal, nutritional and chemical imbalances may contribute to causing the symptoms. Even more confusing for patients and physicians alike is that the underlying causes may differ from one woman to another. Though it is not entirely known what causes the anxiety symptoms, research suggests that several types of imbalances are likely culprits.

One possible cause is an imbalance in the body's estrogen and progesterone levels. Both estrogen and progesterone increase during the second half of the menstrual cycle. Their chemical actions affect the function of almost every organ system in the body. When properly balanced, estrogen and progesterone promote healthy and balanced emotions.

However, PMS mood symptoms may occur if the balance between these hormones is abnormal, because they have an opposing effect on the chemistry of the brain. Estrogen acts as a natural mood elevator and stimulant while progesterone has a sedative effect on the nervous system.

If estrogen predominates, women tend to feel anxious and irritable; and if progesterone predominates, women tend to feel depressed.

Other examples of the opposing effects of estrogen and progesterone include the following: estrogen lowers blood sugar, progesterone elevates it; estrogen promotes synthesis of fats in the tissues, progesterone breaks them down. Thus, when estrogen and progesterone are appropriately balanced, women are more likely to have normal mood and behavioral patterns.

The balance between these hormones depends on two things: how much hormone the body produces, and how efficiently the body breaks it down and disposes of it. The ovaries are the primary source of estrogen and progesterone in premenopausal women (with estrogen also being synthesized by intestinal bacteria and by conversion of adrenal hormones to estrogen by the fatty tissues). The liver has the major responsibility for breaking down and inactivating estrogen. The liver tries to make sure the levels of estrogen circulating through the body in a chemically active form don't become too high.

Breakdown in the liver's ability to perform this function affects the levels of estrogen in the body. Both emotional stress and your nutritional habits play significant roles in how efficiently this system will run. For example, excessive intake of fats, alcohol, and sugar stresses the liver, which must process these foods as well as the hormone.

With vitamin B deficiency, which can be caused by poor nutrition or by emotional stress, the liver lacks the raw material to carry out its metabolic tasks. In either case, the liver cannot break down the hormones efficiently, so higher levels of hormones continue to circulate in the blood without proper disposal, tipping the balance toward excessive anxiety-producing estrogen.

Other research studies link the emotional symptoms of PMS to chemical imbalances in the brain and central nervous system. Some researchers suggest that the symptoms of anxiety and mood swings are due to a heightened sensitivity in some women to fluctuations in the body's level of beta-endorphins. These substances are the body's natural opiates, producing a sense of well-being and even elation when present in large amounts. (Beta endorphins are responsible for the "runner's high" that many people experience after prolonged aerobic exercise, because exercise increases beta endorphin production.)

Beta-endorphin levels increase soon after ovulation at mid-cycle and may decline with the approach of menstruation. A fall in beta-endorphin levels in women who are very sensitive to the effects of these chemicals or who produce large amounts of beta-endorphins could, like opiate withdrawal, cause symptoms such as anxiety and irritability.

Another possible cause of PMS anxiety symptoms may be the lack of sufficient serotonin in the brain. As discussed in the previous chapter, serotonin is a neurotransmitter that regulates rapid eye movement (REM) sleep and appetite. Inadequate levels of serotonin could explain the poor sleep quality with the resultant fatigue, anxiety, and irritability from which some women with PMS suffer.

It could also explain, at least in part, why some women with PMS feel that they have such a difficult time controlling their eating habits and managing their food cravings during the premenstrual time. Serotonin is produced in the body from an amino acid called tryptophan. Tryptophan is an essential amino acid that must be replaced daily through adequate dietary intake since our body cannot manufacture it from other sources. Good sources of tryptophan include almonds, pumpkin seeds, and sesame seeds.

Many factors increase the risk of PMS in susceptible women. PMS occurs most frequently in women over 30, in fact, the most severe symptoms occur in women in their thirties and forties. Women are at high risk when they are under significant emotional stress or if they have poor nutritional habits and don't exercise. Women who are unable to tolerate birth control pills seem to be more likely to suffer PMS, as are women who have had a pregnancy complicated by toxemia. Also, the more children a woman has, the more severe her PMS symptoms.

PMS rarely goes away spontaneously without treatment. My experience is that it gets worse with age. Some of my most uncomfortable patients are women in their middle to late forties who are approaching menopause. These women often feel they have the worst of both life phases as they pass from their reproductive years into menopause. Once the PMS is treated, the accompanying fatigue and mood symptoms clear up. Therapies for PMS are discussed in the self-help section of this book.

Since no single hormonal or chemical imbalance has been linked to PMS, there is no single wonder drug cures PMS, although many drugs have been tested. These include hormones, tranquilizers, antidepressants, and diuretics with varying degrees of success. Luckily, the anxiety and mood swing symptoms of PMS as well as the physical symptoms respond very well to healthful lifestyle changes. In my clinical practice, I have found PMS to be a very treatable problem. I have had great success with my all-natural PMS relief program. A therapeutic diet, the use of nutritional supplements, a stress management program and other self-care therapies are very effective in eliminating PMS symptoms.

## Menopause

Menopause, the end of all menstrual bleeding, occurs for most women between the ages of 48 and 52. However, some women cease menstruating as young as their late thirties or early forties, while others continue to menstruate into their mid-fifties. Anxiety, mood swings, and fatigue often accompany this process as women go through the hormonal changes that lead to the cessation of menstruation.

For most women, the transition to menopause occurs gradually, triggered by a slowdown in the function of their ovaries. The process begins four to six years before the last menstrual period and continues for several years after. During this period of transition, estrogen production from the ovaries decreases, eventually dropping to such low levels that menstruation becomes irregular and finally ceases entirely. For some women this transition to a new, lower level of hormonal equilibrium is easy and uneventful. For many women, however, the transition is difficult, fraught with many uncomfortable symptoms, such as irregular bleeding, hot flashes, anxiety, mood swings, and fatigue. As many as 80 percent of women going through menopause experience some type of mood related symptoms.

In my medical practice, I have also seen many women who experienced marked emotional symptoms while going through menopause. In fact, many of my patients have described symptoms similar to those of PMS. The psychological symptoms of menopause include insomnia (often associated with hot flashes), irritability, anxiety, depression, and fatigue. As mentioned in the section on PMS, both estrogen and progesterone have been studied for their effects on mood: If estrogen predominates, women tend to feel anxious; if progesterone predominates, women may feel depressed and tired.

As women go through menopause, there is first an imbalance in these hormones and finally a deficiency in both as their ovarian production drops to very low levels. The severity of the symptoms probably depends on the individual woman's biochemistry as well as on psychosocial factors. Women have worse symptoms if they are under severe emotional stress or have aggravating dietary habits, such as excessive caffeine, sugar, or alcohol intake.

The emotional symptoms of menopause can also be aggravated by lifestyle issues. For some women, the social and cultural factors occurring before, during, and after menopause may be quite stressful. Menopause can be a time when children leave home and move away, major career changes are made, and marriage ends in divorce or starts anew. Of course, these major life changes can occur at other times besides mid-life but the combination of hormonal and biochemical changes plus lifestyle changes can be quite difficult to handle.

There are many effective treatments to reduce the emotional and physical symptoms of menopause. These include hormonal replacement therapy and, in more severe cases, the use of mood-altering drugs. Vitamins, minerals and herbs can help support a woman's reproductive end endocrine health during menopause. Stress-management techniques and regular exercise may also help restore energy and vitality and stabilize mood. These are discussed in the self-help section of this book.

### Adrenal Stress

The adrenal glands are part of our stress response system. The adrenals are triangular-shaped organs resting on top of each kidney. Each gland consists of two parts, the medulla, or central section, and the cortex, or outer section. Part of the nervous system called the Sympathetic Nervous System (SNS) sends nerve impulses into the adrenal medulla causing it to secrete the same type of chemicals as the sympathetic nerves themselves: the hormones epinephrine (commonly referred to as adrenaline) and norepinephrine (or noradrenaline).

However, while the SNS secretes these chemicals directly into the tissues, the adrenal medulla secretes them into the bloodstream, which transports them to various target tissues, also in response to stressful situations. Thus, the body has two overlapping systems to manage stress: the production of epinephrine and norepinephrine by both the SNS and the adrenal medulla.

The adrenal cortex, or outer portion of the adrenal gland, also produces hormones that help us to manage stress, called mineralocorticoids and glucocorticoids. Adrenal hormones are primarily produced from acetyl Coenzyme A (acetyl CoA) and cholesterol. Acetyl CoA is a chemical produced in the liver, made from fatty acids and amino acids. Cholesterol is a waxy, white, fatty material, widely distributed in all body cells. The cholesterol in the body is supplied by animal foods in the diet, such as eggs and organ meats, and the liver also produces a certain amount of cholesterol.

Glucocorticoids are especially important in allowing an individual to withstand various kinds of stress. The secretion of cortisol accounts for at least 95 percent of adrenal-glucocorticoid activity. Cortisol is the primary stress hormone. In an attempt to buffer the effects of stress, cortisol is released when the body is threatened by extreme conditions such as infection, intense heat or cold, surgery, and any kind of trauma. Cortisol acts as a natural anti-inflammatory when the body is assaulted by infection, a sports injury, arthritis, or allergy. Cortisol also affects carbohydrate and fat metabolism, promoting the conversion of stored sugars and fat into energy.

The mineralocorticoid aldosterone, also produced in the adrenal cortex, has an important role in protecting a person from stress by regulating fluid and electrolyte balance in the body. There must be a correct ratio of sodium and potassium ions inside and outside the cells to maintain normal blood pressure and fluid volume.

When stress is constant and of long duration, the adrenals glands can go into overdrive, always being in a state of arousal and pouring out hormones to deal with stress. In the short term, this can worsen anxiety and stress. Over time, the adrenal glands can become exhausted which leads to chronic fatigue and tiredness.

Following a therapeutic diet, taking beneficial nutritional supplements, managing stress and practicing relaxation techniques are necessary to balance and restore the adrenals. Many helpful self-care treatments listed in the self-care section of this book can help to support the adrenal glands.

## Hyperthyroidism

When the thyroid gland excretes an excessive amount of thyroid hormone, hyperthyroidism occurs. This is a potentially serious and dangerous problem if not diagnosed right away. Symptoms of hyperthyroidism can mimic those of anxiety attacks, and include generalized anxiety, insomnia, easy fatigability, rapid heartbeat, sweating, heat intolerance, and loose bowel movements. In fact, the correct diagnosis may often be missed initially, especially with women who are in menopause, if the symptoms are thought to be due simply to stress or the change of life.

Hyperthyroidism does, however, present with other symptoms that should tip off both the woman and her physician that there is a physiological imbalance present. These symptoms include weight loss despite a ravenous appetite, quick movements, trembling of the hands, and difficulty focusing the eyes.

On a medical examination, many signs of hyperthyroidism may also be present. The skin of a woman with this problem is usually warm and moist. A goiter (enlargement of the thyroid) may be felt by the physician. The skin and hair are usually thin and silky in texture. The eyes usually tend to stare, and in more advanced cases, even bulge from the eye sockets. In advanced cases, there are also muscle wasting and bone loss (osteoporosis) as well as heart abnormalities. As you can see, hyperthyroidism causes severe and potentially dangerous changes in the body and should be considered when trying to diagnose the cause of anxiety episodes.

A diagnosis of hyperthyroidism can be made early by blood tests that show excessive secretion of thyroid hormones, as well as other changes in the blood. If heart and bone abnormalities are present also, they may show on an electrocardiograph and on x-rays. Once diagnosed, hyperthyroidism should be treated immediately to reduce the hormonal output. Treatments include the use of drugs that suppress and even inactivate the thyroid gland, as well as surgical removal of the thyroid. This is discussed in detail in drug chapter of this book.

Women with thyroid dysfunction often have exhaustion in other endocrine glands. The adrenal glands are particularly affected by poor thyroid function, as well as any other physical and emotional stress. The adrenals are two almond-sized glands that secrete several dozen hormones. One of these is cortisol, an important hormone that helps regulate our response to stress. Stress can be a response to strong emotional feelings, such as anxiety or depression, or to physical triggers, such as an allergic reaction, infectious disease, burns, surgery, or an accident. Whatever the source of stress, cortisol lessens its injurious effects on the body, reducing pain, swelling, and fever.

When stress has been recurrent and of long duration, the adrenal glands can become exhausted, providing less and less ability to buffer the negative effects of physical and emotional stress. As a result of adrenal exhaustion, the individual may experience an increase in fatigue and tiredness. Much rest, stress management, and nutritional support are required to restore the adrenals and rebuild the physiological "cushion" to deal with stress. There are many helpful techniques listed in the self-help section of this book to help restore the glandular system.

## Hypoglycemia

This condition occurs when the blood sugar levels in the body fall too low. With this condition, people experience many symptoms similar to those of anxiety and panic attacks. These include anxiety, irritability, trembling, disorientation, light-headedness, spaciness and even palpitations. The dietary trigger for hypoglycemia episodes is excessive intake of simple sugars such as white sugar, soft drinks, fruit juice, white flour products, and sugar-laden desserts such as cookies, doughnuts, and candies.

Glucose, or sugar, is critical for survival because it is the major fuel our bodies run on (the brain alone uses up to 20 percent of the glucose available in the body to fuel its normal level of functioning). However, simple sugars require little processing in the digestive tract and are absorbed rapidly into the blood circulation, overloading the body with fuel. To move this abundance of sugar into the cells where it can be processed and utilized for the cells' energy needs, the hormone insulin is released from the pancreas.

Without adequate insulin, sugar cannot be moved into the cells. When too much sugar is dumped into the blood circulation, usually the reverse situation occurs and too much insulin is secreted. This can actually drop the blood sugar too low (below 70 milligrams per milliliter) to levels where the typical anxiety-like symptoms of hypoglycemia occur. Interestingly, drops in the blood sugar level can also occur simply in response to heightened levels of stress, because the body utilizes extra glucose or fuel during this time.

When the blood sugar level falls too low, the brain is rapidly deprived of energy. A correction must occur in order to bring the glucose levels back to normal, so the adrenal glands release the hormones cortisol and adrenaline that cause the liver to release stored sugar. Though the stored sugar from the liver does restore the blood sugar balance, the rise in adrenal hormonal output also increases emotional arousal and anxiety.

The hypoglycemia cycle can perpetuate the physical and psychological symptoms of anxiety. Women who continue to eat a diet high in simple sugar often feel as though they are on an emotional roller coaster, tossed from highs to lows of anxiety and irritability on the one hand and fatigue and depression on the other, as their blood sugar levels fluctuate.

Most women can easily solve this problem by switching to a diet high in complex carbohydrate foods. These include whole grains, starches, whole fruits, and vegetables. When eaten by themselves or when combined with high-quality proteins and essential fatty acids such as found in nuts, seeds, and fish, the complex carbohydrates are broken down to glucose and slowly absorbed into the blood circulation, thus not triggering excessive insulin output. As a result, both the blood sugar level and the emotions stay healthy and balanced.

In addition, consuming proper vitamins and minerals supports glucose metabolism and pancreatic function, thereby preventing symptoms in women prone to hypoglycemia-related anxiety attacks. Both the optimal diet and nutritional supplements for hypoglycemia are discussed in the self-help chapters of this book.

## Anxiety Due to Immune System Imbalances

Immune system disorders can cause a variety of psychological as well as physical symptoms. These imbalances are discussed in detail in this section.

### Allergies, Including Food Allergies

Many women are unaware that allergic reactions can cause mood changes such as anxiety. Allergies occur when the body's immune system over-reacts to harmless substances. Normally, the immune system is on the alert for invaders such as viruses, bacteria, and other organisms that cause disease. The job of the immune system is to identify these invaders and to produce antibodies that destroy them before they cause illness. In allergic people, this system begins to react to other substances — typically pollens, molds, or foods. Common food allergens include wheat, milk (and milk products), alcohol, chocolate, sugar, eggs, yeast, peanuts, citrus fruits, tomatoes, corn, and shellfish.

Food allergies initiate a series of chemical reactions in the body that include the increase in histamine levels that cause inflammations in tissues where allergic symptoms often appear such as the sinuses, lungs and digestive tract. Sometimes allergic reactions are easily diagnosed, because the symptoms occur immediately after the encounter with the allergen. Immediate allergic symptoms include wheezing, itching and tearing of the eyes, nasal congestion, and hives.

Some allergic reactions, however, are delayed. They may occur hours or days after exposure to the allergen. Delayed symptoms include anxiety, depression, fatigue, dizziness, spaciness, headaches, joint and muscle aches and pains, and eczema. The person affected may be unaware that an allergy is causing her symptoms.

Food allergies can also affect digestive function, causing inflammation of the intestinal lining and pain in the abdominal area. Damage to the intestinal lining causes it to become more porous and permeable. When large particles of poorly digested food, to which the person is allergic, are absorbed into the body, the body's defense system is activated, precipitating damage to many organs and tissues by autoantibodies. (These are the immune complexes that attack your own tissues as if they were foreign substances.) The person affected may be unaware that an allergy is causing her emotional and physical symptoms. This often occurs with food allergies, as well as with a variety of chemical triggers.

Food allergies commonly trigger anxiety episodes in susceptible women. Often, you crave the foods to which you are allergic. Thus, food addiction may actually be a sign of food allergy. Women commonly crave foods such as chocolate, chips, pasta, bread, and milk products. Often they find that once they start eating these foods, they have a difficult time stopping. A woman who has the desire to have one chocolate can end up eating a whole box. The decision to eat one cookie can turn into a binge of ten or fifteen at one session, or a small dish of ice cream becomes a pint.

Though bingeing tendencies can be seen throughout the month in women with food allergies, they tend to be worse during the premenstrual period (which may commence as early as two weeks prior to the onset of menstruation). Alterations in mood as well as physical symptoms typical of anxiety, such as increased heart rate and respiration, often coexist with the food craving symptoms.

Conventional physicians test for food allergies by doing skin tests and blood testing. Unfortunately, these tests are often inaccurate in determining actual food sensitivities. Many people test positively to many healthy foods that they are not allergic to. Some holistic physicians test for food allergies by doing sublingual provocative tests. In this test, a food extract is placed under the tongue to see whether it elicits a reaction. Neutralizing antidotes are then administered to the patient to reduce or eliminate symptoms. This test, however, is not used by traditional allergists.

Finally, there is a blood test called the ELISA (enzyme-linked immune-absorbent assey) that measures the amount of allergen-specific antibodies in your blood. The advantage of allergy blood testing is that it requires only one needle stick, unlike skin testing. However, this test is more expensive and may not be covered by your health insurance.

One of the easiest ways to test for food sensitivities is simply to eliminate suspected food allergens and over the next month or two see what the affect is on your symptoms. Your doctor may ask you to reintroduce these foods one at a time to see how you react. Many women will find that they feel quite a bit better when they eliminate common allergens like gluten-containing grains such as wheat, dairy products, sugar and soy or other foods to which you suspect you may be allergic. Maintaining a low-stress diet can take a load off of the immune system, allowing both your mood and energy to normalize.

During the period when you are determining your food allergies, you may want to keep a diary in which you record your emotional and physical symptoms, both on and off the offending foods, if you try to reintroduce any of them. This will help you evaluate the severity of your reactions.

The conventional treatment for allergy usually includes avoiding the offending substance, if possible, or using over-the-counter and prescription medication and desensitization shots. Alternative health care doctors are also likely to recommend managing stress and following an elimination diet and nutritional supplement program to help treat and prevent allergies. It is important to rotate foods and choose from a wide variety of high-nutrient food. Certain nutritional supplements also help to support and strengthen the immune system. These topics are discussed in the self-care section of this book. Besides avoiding the offending substance, Conventional doctors will recommend the use of prescription and over-the-counter medication and desensitization shots.

## Anxiety Due to Cardiovascular System Disorders

While cardiovascular problems primarily cause physical symptoms, mitral valve prolapse can cause psychological symptoms as well.

### *Mitral Valve Prolapse*

Mitral valve prolapse is a heart condition that can cause anxiety-like episodes of palpitations, chest pain, shortness of breath, and fatigue. It does appear to be present more frequently in people with anxiety and panic episodes than in the general population. It is caused by a mild defect in the mitral valve, which is located between the upper and lower chamber on the left side of the heart. Normally, blood flows unimpeded between the two chambers. However, with mitral valve prolapse, the valve doesn't close completely. As a result, the heart is put under stress and can beat either too fast or erratically. When listening to the heart with a stethoscope, you doctor will often hear a clicking sound that reflects the abnormal changes in the mitral valve. If there is associated leakage (regurgitation) of the blood through the abnormal valve opening, a murmur can also be heard right after the clicking sound.

In more severe cases, the heartbeat can be slowed through the use of beta blockers, drugs that decrease heart rate and heart contractility by decreasing oxygen consumption. (This is discussed in detail in the drug chapter of this book.) In addition, undue stress and stimulants such as caffeine-containing beverages like coffee, tea, and cola drinks should be eliminated in order to avoid triggering episodes of rapid heartbeat. Deficiencies of calcium, magnesium, and potassium should be avoided since these essential minerals help to regulate and reduce cardiac irritability. To ensure adequate daily intake, it is important to maintain a diet with sufficient amounts of these nutrients or to use supplements.

## Common Causes of Anxiety

| Types of anxiety disorders | Physical conditions associated with anxiety | |
|---|---|---|
| Generalized anxiety disorder | Premenstrual syndrome | Hypoglycemia |
| Panic disorder | Menopause | Food allergies |
| Phobias | Hyperthyroidism | Mitral valve prolapse |

# Part II:
# Evaluating Your Symptoms

# 3

## The Anxiety and Stress Workbook

In this chapter, I provide you with a very useful workbook that will assist you in pinpointing the risk factors in your own life that may be contributing to your anxiety and stress symptoms. Many of these questions are similar to the medical history that I take with patients.

I recommend that you fill out the questionnaires in this workbook. They will help you to become aware of possible risk factors that may be triggering your anxiety symptoms based on your lifestyle habits. They will also help you to pinpoint the link between any health problems that you may have and your anxiety symptoms.

The workbook will show you areas in your life that need attention and modification so that you can receive the greatest benefit from the treatment chapters in this book. You can also share this information with your own doctor or health care provider, thereby providing more complete data when a medical exam is performed. I have personally found it very helpful when my patients share the following charts with me.

This workbook section can help you evaluate many of the factors that contribute to anxiety and stress. First, begin to fill out the checklist of anxiety and stress symptoms, starting today. It will be helpful to make several copies of the checklist. If you recall your symptoms for the past month, chart these symptoms as well. The checklist will allow you to see which types of symptoms you have, as well as evaluate their severity. This will make it easier for you to select the specific self-care treatments for symptom relief. Then, as you follow the program, you can keep using the checklists to track your progress.

After you have filled out the checklist, look over the risk factor and lifestyle evaluations that follow. They will help you assess specific areas of your life to see which of your habit patterns may be contributing to your symptoms. Your lifestyle habits are probably significantly impacting the symptoms of anxiety and stress that you are experiencing. By filling out the checklists, you can easily recognize your vulnerable areas. I have also included a chapter on how your doctor or caregiver would likely diagnose the causes of your symptoms from the medical standpoint.

When you've completed these evaluations, you will be ready to go on to the self-help chapters and begin your self-care treatment program.

Grade your symptoms as you experience them each month

*Monthly Calendar of Anxiety and Stress Symptoms*

○ None    ✔ Mild    ◗ Moderate    ● Severe    Date ___

| Symptom / DAY OF CYCLE | 1 | 2 | 3 | 4 | 5 | 6 | 7 | 8 | 9 | 10 | 11 | 12 | 13 | 14 | 15 | 16 | 17 | 18 | 19 | 20 | 21 | 22 | 23 | 24 | 25 | 26 | 27 | 28 | 29 | 30 | 31 |
|---|---|---|---|---|---|---|---|---|---|---|---|---|---|---|---|---|---|---|---|---|---|---|---|---|---|---|---|---|---|---|---|
| Excessive tension or nervousness | | | | | | | | | | | | | | | | | | | | | | | | | | | | | | | |
| Feelings of being on edge | | | | | | | | | | | | | | | | | | | | | | | | | | | | | | | |
| Easily startled, jumpy | | | | | | | | | | | | | | | | | | | | | | | | | | | | | | | |
| Difficulty falling or staying asleep | | | | | | | | | | | | | | | | | | | | | | | | | | | | | | | |
| Easily angered, irritable | | | | | | | | | | | | | | | | | | | | | | | | | | | | | | | |
| Restlessness, easily excited | | | | | | | | | | | | | | | | | | | | | | | | | | | | | | | |
| Dizziness, shakiness, tremulousness | | | | | | | | | | | | | | | | | | | | | | | | | | | | | | | |
| Difficulty concentrating or focusing | | | | | | | | | | | | | | | | | | | | | | | | | | | | | | | |
| Blue moods alternating with anxiety | | | | | | | | | | | | | | | | | | | | | | | | | | | | | | | |
| Excessive tiredness or fatigue | | | | | | | | | | | | | | | | | | | | | | | | | | | | | | | |
| Fear of certain locations, situations | | | | | | | | | | | | | | | | | | | | | | | | | | | | | | | |
| Fear of other people | | | | | | | | | | | | | | | | | | | | | | | | | | | | | | | |
| Frequent nightmares | | | | | | | | | | | | | | | | | | | | | | | | | | | | | | | |
| Muscle tightness or tension | | | | | | | | | | | | | | | | | | | | | | | | | | | | | | | |
| Fast or irregular heartbeat | | | | | | | | | | | | | | | | | | | | | | | | | | | | | | | |
| Chest pain | | | | | | | | | | | | | | | | | | | | | | | | | | | | | | | |
| Shortness of breath | | | | | | | | | | | | | | | | | | | | | | | | | | | | | | | |
| Excessive sweating | | | | | | | | | | | | | | | | | | | | | | | | | | | | | | | |
| Dry mouth | | | | | | | | | | | | | | | | | | | | | | | | | | | | | | | |
| Intestinal cramps, nausea, diarrhea | | | | | | | | | | | | | | | | | | | | | | | | | | | | | | | |
| Frequent urination | | | | | | | | | | | | | | | | | | | | | | | | | | | | | | | |
| Hot flashes or feeling of chilliness | | | | | | | | | | | | | | | | | | | | | | | | | | | | | | | |
| Cold hands and feet | | | | | | | | | | | | | | | | | | | | | | | | | | | | | | | |
| Tightness in throat or lump in throat | | | | | | | | | | | | | | | | | | | | | | | | | | | | | | | |

## Risk Factors for Anxiety

You are at higher risk for developing symptoms of anxiety and stress if you have any of the risk factors listed below. Be sure to follow the exercise, nutritional, and stress management guidelines in the self-care section of this book if you have any of the related risk factors for anxiety listed here. Place a check beside each risk factor that applies to you.

### Risk Factors

| | |
|---|---|
| Relatives with a history of anxiety disorders or phobias | ___ |
| History of overly critical parents, lack of emotional nurturing | ___ |
| History of parents who suppressed and punished and communication and verbalization of feelings | ___ |
| History of fearful and overly cautious parents | ___ |
| History of fearing separation from parents in childhood (going to school, play activities, or even falling asleep without parents) | ___ |
| Significant life stress such as death, illness, or divorce preceding onset of excessive anxiety | ___ |
| PMS | ___ |
| Menopause | ___ |
| Hyperthyroidism (excessive thyroid function) | ___ |
| Hypoglycemia | ___ |
| Food allergies or allergy to food additives | ___ |
| Food addictions | ___ |
| Mitral valve prolapse | ___ |
| Use of estrogen-containing medication | ___ |
| Withdrawal from alcohol, tranquilizers, or sedatives | ___ |
| Use of recreational drugs (such as cocaine, amphetamines) that increase anxiety levels | ___ |

Excessive use of coffee, black tea, colas, chocolates, or other caffeine-containing foods                                                    ____

Excessive use of sugar                                                    ____

Lack of calcium, magnesium, or potassium through insufficient intake of vegetables, fruits, legumes and whole grains in your diet or not using nutritional supplements                                                    ____

Lack of B vitamins in the diet or not using nutritional supplements                                                    ____

## Eating Habits Checklist

Check the number of times you eat the following foods.

### Foods That Increase Symptoms

| Foods | Never | 1x a Month | 1x a Week | >1x a Week |
|---|---|---|---|---|
| Coffee | | | | |
| Cow's milk | | | | |
| Cow's cheese | | | | |
| Butter | | | | |
| Chocolate | | | | |
| Sugar | | | | |
| Alcohol | | | | |
| White bread | | | | |
| White noodles | | | | |
| White-based flour | | | | |
| Pastries | | | | |
| Added salt | | | | |
| Bouillon | | | | |
| Commercial salad dressing, condiments | | | | |
| Coffee | | | | |
| Black tea | | | | |
| Soft drinks | | | | |
| Hot dogs | | | | |
| Ham | | | | |
| Bacon | | | | |
| Beef | | | | |
| Lamb | | | | |
| Pork | | | | |

## Foods That Decrease Symptoms

| | | | | |
|---|---|---|---|---|
| Avocado | | | | |
| Green Beans | | | | |
| Beets | | | | |
| Broccoli | | | | |
| Brussels sprouts | | | | |
| Cabbage | | | | |
| Carrots | | | | |
| Celery | | | | |
| Collard greens | | | | |
| Cucumbers | | | | |
| Eggplant | | | | |
| Garlic | | | | |
| Horseradish | | | | |
| Kale | | | | |
| Legumes | | | | |
| Lettuce | | | | |
| Mustard greens | | | | |
| Okra | | | | |
| Onions | | | | |
| Parsnips | | | | |
| Peas | | | | |
| Potatoes | | | | |
| Radishes | | | | |
| Rutabagas | | | | |
| Spinach | | | | |
| Squash | | | | |
| Sweet potatoes | | | | |
| Tomatoes | | | | |
| Turnips | | | | |
| Turnip greens | | | | |
| Yams | | | | |
| Brown rice | | | | |
| Millet | | | | |
| Barley | | | | |
| Oatmeal | | | | |
| Buckwheat | | | | |
| Raw chia seeds | | | | |
| Raw flaxseeds | | | | |
| Raw tahini | | | | |
| Raw pumpkin seeds | | | | |

| | | | | |
|---|---|---|---|---|
| Raw sesame seeds | | | | |
| Raw sunflower seeds | | | | |
| Raw almonds | | | | |
| Raw filberts | | | | |
| Raw pecans | | | | |
| Raw walnuts | | | | |
| Apples | | | | |
| Bananas | | | | |
| Berries | | | | |
| Pears | | | | |
| Seasonal fruits | | | | |
| Corn oil | | | | |
| Flax oil | | | | |
| Olive oil | | | | |
| Sesame oil | | | | |
| Safflower oil | | | | |
| Eggs | | | | |
| Poultry | | | | |
| Fish | | | | |

## Key to Eating Habits

All the foods listed in the shaded section are unhealthy foods that can increase the symptoms of anxiety and stress. In addition, many of these foods tend to worsen your health in general and should be avoided. If you eat many of these foods, or if you eat any of these foods frequently, your nutritional habits may be contributing significantly to your symptoms. For further guidance on food selection, refer to the chapters on diet, menu planning and recipes.

The foods listed in the unshaded area, from avocados to fish, are high nutrient, low-stress foods that may help relieve or prevent anxiety and stress symptoms. Include these foods frequently in your diet. If you are already eating many of these and very few of the high-stress foods, chances are your nutritional habits are good, and food selection may not be a significant factor in worsening your symptoms.

## Exercise Habits Checklist

Check the frequency with which you do any of the following:

| Activity | Never | 1x a Month | 1 - 2x a Week | >2x a Week |
|---|---|---|---|---|
| Aerobic exercise | | | | |
| Bicycling | | | | |
| Bowling | | | | |
| Croquet | | | | |
| Gardening | | | | |
| Golf | | | | |
| Hiking | | | | |
| Ice skating | | | | |
| Roller skating | | | | |
| Stretching | | | | |
| Swimming | | | | |
| Walking | | | | |
| Weight lifting, small weights | | | | |
| Yoga | | | | |

## Key to Exercise Habits

Moderate aerobic exercise, stretching and yoga performed in a slow relaxed manner help to relieve symptoms of anxiety and stress. They also help to reduce the symptoms of muscular tension that often accompany the emotional distress. If your total number of exercise periods per week is less than three, you probably need to increase your level of physical activity. See the chapter on exercise for recommendations on the types of exercise that would be best suited for you and help reduce your anxiety symptoms.

In contrast, intense anaerobic exercise like fast running and jogging and bodybuilding can actually worsen anxiety and tension because of the speed and intensity with which the exercise is done. It is important not to over exercise when trying to recover from anxiety and panic episodes. Your goal is to learn better habits of relaxation and to restore a sense of peace and calm. You do not want your workouts to be so intense that they are actually worsening your stress and panic symptoms. If you suspect that this is what is happening to you, you may want to modify your current regimen. You will find many options available in the chapters on physical exercise, stretches, and acupressure.

### Key to Lack of Physical Fitness and Stamina

If you find that symptoms listed in this evaluation pertain to you, you should start a physical fitness program slowly and carefully. Your level of physical activity should be increased gradually until your body is more conditioned to the point where exercise is not as difficult to do. You may want to notify your physician regarding these symptoms. Your physician may then help guide you in designing the best exercise regimen for your needs. In addition, some of these symptoms may indicate an underlying health problem that should be evaluated.

## Symptoms of Lack of Physical Fitness and Stamina

Check those symptoms that pertain to you:

|  | Yes | No |
|---|---|---|
| Fatigue, tiredness, lethargy | —— | —— |
| Tiredness or exhaustion when walking less than a mile | —— | —— |
| Shortness of breath when walking less than a mile | —— | —— |
| Tiredness or exhaustion when walking up a flight of stairs | —— | —— |
| Shortness of breath when walking up a flight of stairs | —— | —— |
| Excessive weight or obesity | —— | —— |
| Poor muscle tone | —— | —— |
| Excessive muscle tension and/or cramping when engaging in physical activity | —— | —— |
| Eyestrain | —— | —— |
| Chronic neck pain and muscle tension | —— | —— |
| Chronic shoulder and upper-middle-back tension | —— | —— |
| Grinding of teeth (bruxism) | —— | —— |
| Chronic low back pain | —— | —— |
| Chronic abdominal tension | —— | —— |
| Chronic arm tension | —— | —— |

## *Key to Daily Exercise Diary*

The following diary should help you determine if your current exercise program is right for helping reduce your anxiety and stress symptoms as well as promote optimal physical conditioning. A good exercise program should leave you feeling energized and relaxed at the same time. You should also do activities you enjoy so that you look forward to your exercise session.

If, when filling out the diary, you find that your exercise program is not satisfactory, then switch to other physical activities. Read the chapters on physical exercise, stretches, and acupressure massage for other options.

## Daily Exercise Diary

Month_____

| | Date | Time | Exercise type | Session length | Pulse rate |
|---|---|---|---|---|---|
| 1 | | | | | |
| 2 | | | | | |
| 3 | | | | | |
| 4 | | | | | |
| 5 | | | | | |
| 6 | | | | | |
| 7 | | | | | |
| 8 | | | | | |
| 9 | | | | | |
| 10 | | | | | |
| 11 | | | | | |
| 12 | | | | | |
| 13 | | | | | |
| 14 | | | | | |
| 15 | | | | | |
| 16 | | | | | |
| 17 | | | | | |
| 18 | | | | | |
| 19 | | | | | |
| 20 | | | | | |
| 21 | | | | | |
| 22 | | | | | |
| 23 | | | | | |
| 24 | | | | | |
| 25 | | | | | |
| 26 | | | | | |
| 27 | | | | | |
| 28 | | | | | |
| 29 | | | | | |
| 30 | | | | | |
| 31 | | | | | |

## **Responses**
Emotional

## **Responses**
Physical

1 _____  _____
2 _____  _____
3 _____  _____
4 _____  _____
5 _____  _____
6 _____  _____
7 _____  _____
8 _____  _____
9 _____  _____
10 _____  _____
11 _____  _____
12 _____  _____
13 _____  _____
14 _____  _____
15 _____  _____
16 _____  _____
17 _____  _____
18 _____  _____
19 _____  _____
20 _____  _____
21 _____  _____
22 _____  _____
23 _____  _____
24 _____  _____
25 _____  _____
26 _____  _____
27 _____  _____
28 _____  _____
29 _____  _____
30 _____  _____
31 _____  _____

## Major Life Stress Evaluation

Major life stress can have a significant impact on the emotional symptoms of anxiety and nervous tension as well as on other health problems linked to these symptoms. It is helpful to assess your own level of stress to see how it may be impacting your health. One popular tool is the Holmes and Rahe Social Readjustment Rating Scale that I have adapted for women and identifies events that cause stress.

Check those life events that pertain to you. This will help you evaluate the level of major stress in your life.

_____ Death of spouse or close family member

_____ Divorce from spouse

_____ Death of a close friend

_____ Legal separation from spouse

_____ Loss of job

_____ Radical loss of financial security

_____ Major personal injury or illness (gynecologic or other cause)

_____ Future surgery for gynecologic or other illness

_____ Beginning a new marriage

_____ Foreclosure of mortgage or loan

_____ Lawsuit lodged against you

_____ Marriage reconciliation

_____ Change in health of a family member

_____ Major trouble with boss or co-workers

_____ Increase in responsibility—job or home

_____ Learning you are pregnant

_____ Difficulties with your sexual abilities

_____ Gaining a new family member

_____ Change to a different job

_____ Increase in number of marital arguments

_____ New loan or mortgage of more than $100,000

_____ Son or daughter leaving home

_____ Major disagreement with in-laws or friends

_____ Recognition for outstanding achievements

_____ Spouse begins or stops work

_____ Begin or end education

_____ Undergo a change in living conditions

_____ Revise or alter your personal habits

_____ Change in work hours or conditions

_____ Change of residence

_____ Change your school or major in school

_____ Alterations in your recreational activities

_____ Change in church or club activities

_____ Change in social activities

_____ Change in sleeping habits

_____ Change in number of family get-togethers

_____ Diet or eating habits are changed

_____ You go on vacation

_____ The year-end holidays occur

_____ You commit a minor violation of the law

## Key to Major Life Stress Evaluation

Checking many items in the first third of this scale indicates major life stress and a possible vulnerability to serious illness. As you go down the list, the stresses decrease in the degree to which they cause major emotional dislocation. For example, a death or divorce is much more traumatic for most people than changing their school or major, if you are a student. Thus, the more items checked in the first third of the scale, the higher your stress quotient.

Do everything possible to manage your stress in a healthy way. Eat the foods that provide a high-nutrient/low-stress diet, do moderate aerobic exercise on a regular basis, and learn the methods for managing stress given in the chapters on renewing your mind, meditation and deep breathing exercises.

If you check fewer items, you are probably at lower risk for illness. Because stresses too minimal to include in this evaluation may also play a part in increasing your level of anxiety and nervous tension, you will still benefit from practicing the methods outlined in the chapter on stress reduction. Stress management is very important in helping you reduce your symptoms of anxiety and panic attacks as well as your level of muscle tension.

## Daily Stress Evaluation

This evaluation is very important for women with anxiety. Not all stresses have as major an impact in our lives. Most of us are exposed to a multitude of small life stresses on a daily basis. In filling out this questionnaire, you may find a number of stresses that are triggering emotional upset and anxiety in your life. In addition, the effects of these stresses can be cumulative. They can be a major factor in creating chronic wear and tear on our immune, endocrine and circulatory systems. In addition, daily stress often triggers chronic muscle tension and pain. Check each item that seems to apply to you.

### Work

____ **Too much responsibility.** You feel you have to push too hard to do your work. There are too many demands made of you. You feel very pressured by all of this responsibility. You worry about getting all your work done and doing it well.

____ **Time urgency.** You worry about getting your work done on time. You always feel rushed. It feels like there are not enough hours in the day to complete your work.

____ **Job instability.** You are concerned about losing your job. There are layoffs at your company. There is much insecurity and concern among your fellow employees about their job security.

____ **Job performance.** You don't feel that you are working up to your maximum capability due to outside pressures or stress. You are unhappy with your job performance and concerned about job security as a result.

____ **Difficulty getting along with co-workers and boss.** Your boss is too picky and critical. Your boss demands too much. You must work closely with co-workers who are difficult to get along with.

____ **Understimulation.** Work is boring. The lack of stimulation makes you tired. You wish you were somewhere else.

____ **Uncomfortable physical plant.** Noises are too loud. You are exposed to noxious fumes or chemicals. There is too much activity going on around you, making it difficult to concentrate.

## Home

____ **Home organization.** Home is poorly organized. It always seems messy; chores are half-finished. You feel tense and stressed while in your own home due to the physical disorder.

____ **Time.** There is too much to do in the home and never enough time to get it all done.

____ **Too much responsibility.** You need more help. There are too many demands on your time and energy. You feel tense and anxious as a result

## Spouse or Significant Other

____ **Negative communication.** There is too much negative emotion and drama. You are always upset and angry. There is not enough peace and quiet.

____ **Not enough communication.** There is not enough discussion of feelings or issues. You both tend to hold in your feelings. You feel that an emotional bond is lacking between you.

____ **Discrepancy in communication.** One person talks about feelings too much, the other person too little.

____ **Affection.** You do not feel you receive enough affection. There is not enough holding, touching, and loving in your relationship. Or, you are made uncomfortable by your partner's demands.

____ **Sexuality.** There is not enough sexual intimacy. You feel deprived by your partner. Or, your partner demands sexual relations too often. You feel pressured.

____ **Children.** They make too much noise. They make too many demands on your time. They are hard to discipline.

____ **Organization.** Home is poorly organized. It always seems messy; chores are half-finished.

____ **Time.** There is too much to do in the home and never enough time to get it all done.

____ **Responsibility.** You need more help. There are too many demands on your time and energy.

**Your Emotional State**

____ **Too much anxiety.** You worry too much about every little thing. You constantly worry about what can go wrong in your life.

____ **Victimization.** Everyone is taking advantage of you or wants to hurt you.

____ **Poor self-image.** You don't like yourself enough. You are always finding fault with yourself.

____ **Too critical.** You are always finding fault with others. You always look at what is wrong with other people rather than seeing their virtues.

____ **Inability to relax.** You are always wound up. It is difficult for you to relax. You are tense and restless.

____ **Not enough self-renewal.** You don't play enough or take enough time off to relax and have fun. Life isn't fun and enjoyable as a result.

____ **Feeling of depression.** You feel blue, isolated, and tearful. You feel a sense of self-blame and hopelessness. Fatigue and low energy are problems.

____ **Too angry.** Small life issues seem to upset you unduly. You find yourself becoming angry and irritable with your husband, children, or clients.


## Key to Daily Stress Evaluation

Read over the day-to-day stress areas that you find difficult to handle. Becoming aware of them is the first step toward lessening their effects on your life. Methods for reducing stresses and helping your body to deal with them are given in the chapters on renewing your mind, stress reduction, breathing exercises, stretches and acupressure.

In the next chapter, I want to share with you important information on the steps that your doctor or caregiver is likely to take in diagnosing your symptoms of anxiety and panic attacks from the medical point of view.

# 4

## Diagnosis of Anxiety and Panic Attacks

It is very important to consult with a physician or other caregiver to have an accurate diagnosis of the causes of your anxiety, panic episodes and stress symptoms. Even if you choose to follow a totally all natural treatment program like the one that I share with you in this book, it is still important for your symptoms to be properly evaluated.

Of primary importance is for your physician or caregiver to determine if your symptoms are emotional and psychological in origin or if there are physical causes for your anxiety or panic episodes that need to be corrected.

There are three steps that your physician or caregiver may need to take in order to accurately diagnose anxiety and stress symptoms. This includes taking a medical history, doing a physical examination and then ordering or performing diagnostic tests to better evaluate your condition. This can include doing a variety of blood, saliva or urine tests that seem to be most appropriate to your set of signs and symptoms.

I am going to describe the process of diagnosing anxiety and panic attacks in some detail so that you can know what to expect once you start this process with your own doctor or caregiver.

Let's look now at each of these steps. If you have not already done so, I recommend that you fill out the workbook section questionnaires on your current diet, stress triggers, exercise habits, patterns of muscle tension and other risk factors. You may want to share your responses to these questionnaires with your health care provider because they can offer valuable clues to help discover a medical problem that hasn't yet been diagnosed. Also, be sure to let your physician know if you have any previously diagnosed problems such as mitral valve prolapse, which can also trigger anxiety-like episodes.

## Medical History

Your doctor will begin the process of evaluating the cause of anxiety and panic attacks by taking a careful medical history. You will probably be asked about your symptoms and how they are affecting your mood and body. There are quite a number of symptoms that have been linked to anxiety including being easily startled or feeling jumpy, constant fear or worry that is interfering with your daily life, irritability and restlessness. You may have shortness of breath, chest tightness, pounding of the heart or racing pulse. Other symptoms include frequent urination, diarrhea, upset stomach, excessive sweating, muscle tension, cold hands and feet, headaches, fatigue, and insomnia, or difficulty falling asleep and staying asleep. Your doctor should ask you about many of these symptoms to determine your pattern of stress.

Your caregiver should ask you when you first noticed these symptoms, how often you have anxiety and panic episodes and are there any specific triggers that you are aware of such as being at social gathering, doing public speaking or communicating with your spouse or a family member about sensitive issues that seems to set off these symptoms. It is also important to ask about your diet and if the ingestion of certain foods triggers anxiety episodes. Also, information about the use of nutritional supplements and medications and hormonal therapies such as birth control pills or hormone replacement therapy (HRT) that may be affecting your symptoms should be asked about. Your doctor should find out if the symptoms are related to the timing of your menstrual periods or began to occur with the onset of menopause. This can suggest a possible hormonal trigger for your symptoms.

Risk factors such as dietary and nutritional status and level of personal, work and family stress, as well as drug, alcohol, food and substance abuse or if other family members also suffer from anxiety and panic attacks should also be evaluated. These essential lifestyle factors can significantly affect your level of anxiety and stress. Unfortunately, many of these factors are more likely to be looked at and evaluated by an alternative health practitioner rather than a conventional medical doctor.

## Physical Examination

Your doctor should check your blood pressure and pulse rate to see if stress is causing an elevation in your blood pressure or causing a too rapid pulse rate. He or she should also listen to your heart and lungs to check for abnormalities of the heart rate and rhythm as well as the presence of heart murmurs or abnormal heart sounds.

Women with a heart condition called mitral value prolapse in which the mitral valve prolapse doesn't close properly can cause anxiety-like symptoms as does a condition called paroxysmal supraventricular tachycardia. Mitral valve prolapse can cause a clicking sound that your doctor may hear when listening to your heart with a stethoscope. If there is associated leakage (regurgitation) of the blood through the abnormal valve opening, a murmur can also be heard right after the clicking sound. Lung conditions, such as asthma, that are triggered by stress also need to be listened for and evaluated at this time.

A potentially serious condition that can be overlooked or misdiagnosed is hyperthyroidism. This is particularly true with women in menopause, if the symptoms are thought to be due simply to stress or the change of life. Physical signs of this condition that can be seen on physical examination include warm and moist skin, thin hair, trembling of the hands and enlargement of the thyroid gland that can be felt by your doctor when examining your neck. The eyes may tend to stare and, in more advanced cases, even bulge from the eye sockets.

## Laboratory Testing

Depending on your age, a complete blood count and chemistry panel, urinalysis, blood sugar, thyroid, and hormone panels are frequently used when screening for anxiety. Depending on your medical history and physical examination, other tests may be ordered, also.

Your doctor may choose to have testing of your neurotransmitter levels done. Other tests that may be ordered depending on your symptoms can include allergy testing, testing for adrenal and digestive function and a hormonal panel. If you don't understand any terms or tests used, ask your physician for more information. An informed and educated woman can do a much better job planning and participating in her own wellness program. Let's now look at the different types of testing that may be done.

Brain chemistry testing is somewhat controversial. Some physicians believe strongly in the value of this type of testing to assist in the diagnosis of anxiety and help to select the most effective therapies, especially the amino acids, vitamins and minerals necessary to manufacture neurotransmitters within your body. In contrast, other practitioners think that that these tests are worthless and do not order them. The feelings on this issue can run very strongly from one practitioner to another.

The laboratories that do urine neurotransmitter testing are, in fact, testing the levels of neurotransmitters within the whole body, rather than specifically the brain levels of these chemicals. However, the laboratories that run these tests have correlated the levels of these neurotransmitters with specific psychiatric abnormalities like anxiety.

One such laboratory, NeuroScience, Inc., (888342-7272 or www.neurorelief com) is a leader in the development of neurotransmitter testing. They have developed sensitive testing for these neurochemicals that can be done through your urine. The test is simple to do, noninvasive, and can be done in the privacy of your own home. In addition to NeuroScience, there are many other similar laboratories that offer neurotransmitter testing.

If food addiction to sugar is triggering anxiety symptoms, this may show up when testing your blood sugar level. When too much sugar is dumped into the blood circulation, too much insulin may be secreted. This can actually drop the blood sugar too low (below 70 milligrams per milliliter) to levels where the typical anxiety-like symptoms of hypoglycemia occur. Interestingly, drops in the blood sugar level can also occur simply in response to heightened levels of stress, because the body utilizes extra glucose or fuel during this time.

The diagnosis of hyperthyroidism is confirmed with blood tests that measure the level of your main thyroid hormone, thyroxine, and TSH (thyroid stimulating hormone) produced by the pituitary gland. With this condition, thyroxine levels are too high and your TSH levels are too low. TSH levels are usually elevated in order to send a signal to your thyroid gland to produce more hormones. With hyperthyroidism, this is obviously not necessary since you are actually overproducing thyroid hormone.

Your doctor may also order a thyroid scan during which a radioactive isotope is injected into the vein inside your elbow or hand. This will help to produce an image of your thyroid gland. Another test that may be ordered is the radioactive iodine uptake test. For this test, you are given a small, oral dose of radioactive iodine. This iodine will collect in your thyroid gland since it uses iodine to make thyroid hormone. If you have a high uptake of radioiodine, it indicates that your thyroid gland is producing too much thyroxine.

Conventional physicians usually test for food allergies by doing skin tests and blood testing. Unfortunately, these tests are often inaccurate in determining actual food sensitivities. Many people test positively to many healthy foods that they are not allergic to. Some holistic physicians test for food allergies by doing sublingual provocative tests. In this test, a food extract is placed under the tongue to see whether it elicits a reaction. Neutralizing antidotes are then administered to the patient to reduce or eliminate symptoms. This test, however, is not used by traditional allergists.

Finally, there is a blood test called the ELISA (enzyme-linked immunoabsorbent assey) that measures the amount of allergen-specific antibodies in your blood. The advantage of allergy blood testing is that it requires only one needle stick (unlike skin testing). However, these tests are more expensive and may not be covered by your health insurance.

Testing of adrenal function as a cause of anxiety and panic attacks is difficult to diagnose by traditional blood testing. This is because conventional doctors are looking for more extreme states of adrenal failure (Addison's Disease) or hyperactivity. Alternative medical doctors are more likely to do blood, urine and saliva tests to determine less extreme levels of adrenal stress that may be causing your symptoms. Your doctor may want to tests levels of adrenal hormones and chemicals including cortisol, DHEA, norepinephrine and epinephrine that can help to indicate adrenal function.

If you have symptoms of irritable bowel syndrome, cramping, diarrhea and bloating that is caused by anxiety and stress, your doctor may want to evaluate your digestive function to rule out other causes of these symptoms. These include bacterial, yeast and parasite infections, allergies to common foods like wheat, milk, soy and eggs, deficient enzyme production within the digestive tract and any signs of intestinal bleeding. This can be readily tested with a stool sample that is then sent to the laboratory for analysis.

Besides listening to your heart, mitral valve prolapse can de detected by doing an echocardiogram. An echocardiogram is a noninvasive, ultrasound evaluation of your heart. With this test, high-frequency sound waves are used to create images of your heart and its structures. The valves of your heart can by seen as well as how well the blood is flowing through them. With mitral valve prolapse, this test can measure the severity of the prolapse as well as any associated leakage. Since abnormally rapid or irregular heart rhythms can occur with mitral valve prolapse, your doctor may also order a 24-hour Holter monitor. This device takes a continuous recording of your heart activity as you carry on with your daily activities in order to detect any abnormal heart rhythms.

If your doctor suspects that either PMS or menopause are the cause of your anxiety symptoms, he or she may want to order hormone testing. Until the 1990's, the method for checking women's hormone levels had severe limitations. A single blood sample was taken and analyzed, though the results of this one-time check were unhelpful, given the ebb and flow of your hormone levels throughout the month In addition, the stress of having blood drawn was enough to throw off a woman's hormone levels and skew the results.

Fortunately, female hormone testing done through saliva samples are also now commonly available. Saliva testing is not only non-invasive (no needle sticks!), but it is also highly accurate. These tests can help to evaluate your hormonal status and assist in the design of a treatment program individualized for your anxiety symptoms that can deliver the maximum benefits with minimum risk of side effects.

Best of all, saliva hormone testing is accessible. Even physicians who still don't routinely order saliva hormone testing will usually do so if a patient requests it. You can even order a limited saliva hormone testing kit on your own directly from a laboratory, without a doctor's prescription.

Like blood, saliva closely mirrors hormone levels in your body's tissues. However, saliva is a particularly accurate indicator of free (unbound) hormone levels. This is the key, as only free hormones are active, meaning that they can affect the hormone-sensitive tissues in your breasts, brain, heart, and uterus. Saliva testing therefore provides a superior measure of the levels of hormones that actually affect vital body systems, mood, tissue levels of sodium and fluid, and many other important functions.

Additionally, blood testing only provides a one-time "snapshot" of hormone levels, whereas saliva testing provides a dynamic picture of hormonal ebb and flow over an entire menstrual cycle. In fact, saliva samples are collected during the month, all at the same time of day, and then sent to a laboratory. The lab measures and charts your progesterone and estradiol (your most prevalent and potent form of estrogen) levels. These results are compared to normal patterns. Finally, saliva testing is easy, stress-free and non-invasive. You can collect your own saliva samples, which means you don't have to go to your doctor's office or a lab. Plus, there's no need to draw blood.

If you think saliva hormone testing is right for you, consider consulting your physician. Having your doctor order the test has two advantages: The profile is more extensive, and your insurance may cover the cost. A number of laboratories perform the test. If your doctor doesn't order the test, or you simply want insight to help you develop your own self-care regimen, you can order a test kit from laboratories through the Internet.

Once a definitive diagnosis of anxiety and stress is made, whether psychological or physical, effective treatment can then be instituted to relieve the symptoms and restore your mood and emotional balance. For more details, refer to the treatment sections of this book in which I share my very effective treatment program as well as the most up-to-date information on medical therapies.

# Part III:
# Finding the Solution

# 5

# My Diet for Relief of Anxiety and Stress

In this chapter, I would like to share with you important information about the crucial role that food selection plays in reducing or intensifying your symptoms of anxiety, panic and excessive stress. I have seen this connection with many of my own patients and it has been confirmed by medical research. In fact, the antianxiety diet that I have created for my patients is one of the cornerstones of my self-care program

Many important studies in the field of diet and nutrition over the past few decades have corroborated that certain foods, beverages and food additives can actually worsen or trigger anxiety feelings in women. This is true in emotionally-based as well as chemically or hormonally-based cases of anxiety and panic. Happily, research studies have also found certain foods to be beneficial for their mood-stabilizing and calming properties. Thus, your food selection plays an important role in how well you heal from the anxiety and panic symptoms.

In my practice, I have been thrilled by the benefits of the antianxiety diet for my patients and how well it relieves needless suffering. I have seen thousands of women struggling with anxiety symptoms, due to many different emotional and physical causes, significantly improve when they changed their diets.

A therapeutic diet is an essential part of the treatment program for anxiety caused by brain chemistry imbalances, PMS, hypoglycemia, food allergies as well as other causes. The use of an antianxiety diet can play a major supporting role in reducing unpleasant stress symptoms. In fact, I have found that continuing stressful eating habits can work against other therapeutic measures a patient may institute, such as counseling or the use of antianxiety medication. Thus, the importance of healthful dietary practices in the treatment of anxiety and panic attacks should not be underestimated.

In this chapter, I list and discuss in detail the foods that worsen anxiety and should be avoided. The list may surprise you because it contains foods that are considered staples of the American diet. Many women with anxiety unwittingly eat a diet that worsens their symptoms. I also discuss foods that can improve and enhance your emotional well-being as well as your general state of health. This information is based on successfully assisting thousands of patients who suffered from anxiety and noted significant relief of their symptoms when following this program. It is also based on the medical research in this field.

## Foods to Avoid

It is important to eliminate all foods that intensify your anxiety symptoms. These include foods that are toxic and stressful to the body when used in excess, and that may trigger anxiety symptoms in susceptible women when used even in small amounts. In my experience with patients suffering from moderate to severe anxiety, all of these foods should be entirely eliminated or at least sharply curtailed to small amounts, used on an occasional basis as a treat.

Some women may find that they need to eliminate anxiety-causing foods gradually because of their emotional or physical attachments to the food. When there are strong emotional attachments, the elimination process itself can cause stress; thus, it should be done gently. Many other women find that the "cold turkey" approach works best, and they appreciate the rapid relief from anxiety symptoms that simply eliminating a stressful food brings. I will mention any pitfalls of such an approach when discussing the specific foods in this section.

### Sugar

Glucose, a simple form of sugar, is the food that provides the body with its main source of energy. Without a steady supply of glucose, we could not produce the hundreds of thousands of chemical reactions our bodies need to perform daily functions. The brain is one of the primary users of glucose, requiring 20 percent of the total available glucose to function optimally. However, the form in which you take this important food into your body can affect your mood in a profound manner.

The ideal approach is to eat lots of complex carbohydrates such as whole grains, potatoes, fruit, and vegetables. The sugar in these foods digests slowly and is released into the blood circulation very gradually. Thus, the amount of sugar released from these foods does not overwhelm the body's ability to handle it. Unfortunately, many Americans obtain their sugar intake through the excessive use of simple sugar—the refined white or brown sugar that is the primary ingredient of most cookies, candies, cakes, pies, soft drinks, ice cream, and other sweet foods.

In addition, pasta and bread made from white flour, which has all the bran, essential fatty acids, and nutrients removed, act as simple sugars; unfortunately, these make up a significant part of the diet of many women in Western societies. Many convenience foods, including salad dressing, ketchup, and relish, also contain high levels of both sugar and salt. With sugar so prevalent in many foods, sugar addiction is common in our society among people of all ages. Many people use sweet foods as a way to deal with their frustrations and other upsets. As a result, most Americans consume too much sugar—the average American eats 120 pounds per year.

This excessive level of sugar intake can be a major trigger for anxiety symptoms. Here is what happens: Unlike complex carbohydrates, foods based on sugar and white flour break down quickly in the digestive tract. Glucose is released rapidly into the blood circulation and from there is absorbed by the cells of the body to satisfy their energy needs. To handle this overload, the pancreas must release large amounts of insulin, a chemical that helps move the glucose from the blood circulation into the cells.

Often the pancreas tends to overshoot the amount of insulin needed. As a result, the blood sugar level goes from too high to too low, resulting in the roller coaster effect typically seen in hypoglycemia or PMS. You may initially feel "high" after eating sugar, and then experience a rapid crash and a dip in your energy level. (Excessive amounts of stress also use up glucose rapidly and can cause similar symptoms.)

When your blood sugar level falls too low, you begin to feel anxious, jittery, spacey, and confused because your brain is deprived of its necessary fuel. To remedy this situation, the adrenal glands release cortisol and other hormones that cause your liver to release stored sugar so that your blood sugar can return to normal levels. Though the adrenal hormones boost the blood sugar level, they unfortunately increase arousal symptoms and anxiety too. Thus, both the initial glucose deprivation in the brain and the adrenal's response to restore the glucose levels can intensify symptoms of anxiety and panic in susceptible women.

Excessive use of sugar has further detrimental effects. Like caffeine, sugar depletes the body's B-complex vitamins and minerals, thereby increasing nervous tension, anxiety, and irritability. Too much sugar also intensifies fatigue by narrowing the diameter of the blood vessels and putting stress on the nervous system. Candida feeds on sugar, so overindulging in this high-stress food worsens chronic candida infections. Many women with chronic candida complain of emotional symptoms like depression and nervous tension. Furthermore, sugar (as well as caffeine, alcohol, flavor enhancers, and white flour) appears to be an important trigger for the binge eating often seen with anxiety and PMS.

Research studies have shown that when women switch from a diet high in sugar to a refined sugar free, high-nutrient diet, food addictive behavior tends to cease. After making the switch from a high sugar intake diet, women tend to lose or maintain weight more easily and to successfully maintain relief from the pattern of craving and binging (for up to two years, in one study).

In summary, sugar stresses many bodily systems, worsens your health, and intensifies anxiety, nervous tension, and fatigue. Try to satisfy your sweet tooth instead with healthier foods. Consider fruit or grain-based desserts, like oatmeal cookies sweetened with fruit or honey. You will find that small amounts of these foods can satisfy your cravings. Instead of disrupting your mood and energy level, they actually have a healthful and balancing effect.

## Dairy Products

Women with anxiety and stress symptoms should avoid dairy products. This always surprises women, because dairy products have traditionally been touted as one of the four basic food groups; many women count them as staples in their diet, eating large amounts of cheese, yogurt, milk, and cottage cheese. Yet dairy products are extremely difficult for the body to digest. They can worsen the depression and fatigue that coexist in many women with anxiety symptoms. This is because the body must use so much energy to break them down before they can be absorbed, assimilated, and finally utilized.

All parts of dairy products are difficult to digest—the fat, the protein, and the milk sugar. Digesting dairy products demands hydrochloric acids, enzymes, and fat emulsifiers, which a stressed and tired woman may not produce in sufficient quantities. Many women are specifically allergic to dairy products, and dairy products also intensify allergy symptoms in general. Besides physical symptoms, food allergies can trigger anxiety, mood swings, and even fatigue in susceptible women.

I see this often in my patients who have emotionally-based anxiety symptoms or PMS-related anxiety coexisting with food allergies. Users of dairy products often complain of allergy-based nasal congestion, sinus swelling, and postnasal drip. They can also suffer from digestive problems such as bloating, gas, and bowel changes, which intensify with menstruation. Intolerance to dairy products can hamper the absorption and assimilation of calcium, an important anxiety-relieving mineral.

Dairy products have many other unhealthy effects on a woman's body. The saturated fats in dairy products put women at higher risk of heart disease and cancer of the breast, uterus, and ovaries. Women on a high-fat diet also tend to accumulate excess weight more easily. Many dairy products, such as cheese, are high in salt as well as fat. Excessive use of these foods can increase the risk of high blood pressure and of bloating and fluid retention. Bloating can cause uncomfortable breast tenderness and abdominal swelling, particularly in the premenstrual period.

Women who have depended on dairy products for their calcium intake naturally wonder what alternative sources they should use. Women concerned about calcium intake can turn to many other good dietary sources of this essential nutrient, including beans, peas, soybeans, sesame seeds, soup stock made from chicken or fish bones, and green leafy vegetables. For food preparation, rice, almond, flaxseed, sunflower seed, hempseed, multi-grain and soy milk are excellent substitutes. These nondairy milks are readily available at health food stores. You can also use a supplement containing calcium, vitamin D and magnesium to make sure your intake of these nutrients is sufficient.

## Caffeine

Coffee, black tea, soft drinks, and chocolate all contain caffeine. Many women with anxiety and high stress levels mistakenly use caffeine as a pick-me-up to help them get through the day's tasks. Unfortunately, caffeine can trigger and aggravate anxiety and panic episodes. Caffeine used in excess (more than four or five cups per day) can dramatically increase anxiety, irritability, and mood swings. Even small amounts can make susceptible women jittery. After the initial pick-up, women with anxiety coexisting with excessive stress find that caffeine intake makes them more tired than before.

Caffeine triggers anxiety symptoms because it directly stimulates several arousal mechanisms in the body. It increases the brain's level of norepinephrine, a neurotransmitter that increases alertness. However, it also triggers sympathetic nervous system activity, which causes the fight-or-flight physiological responses in the body, such as increased pulse, breathing rate, and muscle tension. Thus, caffeine intake triggers the physiological responses typical of anxiety states. Caffeine stimulates the release of stress hormones from the adrenal glands, further intensifying symptoms of nervousness and jitteriness.

Caffeine depletes the body's stores of B-complex vitamins and essential minerals, such as potassium, which are important in the chemical reactions that convert food to usable energy. Deficiency of these nutrients increases anxiety, mood swings, and fatigue. Depletion of B-complex vitamins also interferes with carbohydrate metabolism and healthy liver function, which help to regulate the blood sugar as well as estrogen levels. An imbalance in estrogen and progesterone can increase anxiety and mood swings in women with symptoms of PMS or menopause. Many menopausal women also complain that caffeine increases the frequency of hot flashes. Coffee, black tea, chocolate, and soft drinks all act to inhibit iron absorption, thus worsening anemia.

If you suffer from moderate to severe anxiety symptoms due to any cause, I recommend that you reduce your caffeine consumption to one cup of coffee per day and try to eliminate cola drinks, caffeine-containing tea, and chocolate. Some women may find that going "cold turkey" with coffee and eliminating it abruptly causes unpleasant withdrawal symptoms such as headaches, depression, and fatigue. In these cases, it is better to cut down coffee intake gradually, decreasing the amounts slowly over a period of one month to several months, substituting first decaffeinated coffee and finally herbal teas. Many herbal teas, like chamomile and peppermint, even have a relaxant effect on the body, thereby helping to reduce anxiety.

## Caffeine Content of Beverages and Foods
(listed in order of caffeine content)

| Product | Caffeine per Serving |
|---|---|
| Coffee (per cup) | |
|   Drip (average) | 146 mg |
|   Percolated (average) | 110 mg |
| Coffee — instant (per cup) | |
|   Folgers | 97.5 mg |
|   Maxwell House | 94 mg |
|   Nescafe | 81 mg |
| Decaffeinated Coffee (per cup) | |
|   Taster's Choice | 3.5 mg |
| Tea (per cup) | |
|   Tetley | 63.5 mg |
|   Lipton | 52 mg |
|   Constant Comment | 29 mg |
|   Green Tea | 24-40 mg |
| Soft Drinks (per 12 oz. can) | |
|   Mountain Dew | 55 mg |
|   Diet Dr. Pepper | 54 mg |
|   Coke Classic | 46 mg |
|   Diet Coke | 46 mg |
|   Pepsi | 38.4 mg |
|   Diet Pepsi | 36 mg |
| Hot Chocolate Drinks (per cup) | |
|   Cocoa | 13 mg |
| Candy (per oz.) | |
|   Ghirardelli Dark Chocolate | 24 mg |
|   Hershey's Milk Chocolate | 4 mg |

## Alcohol

Women with moderate to severe anxiety and mood swings should avoid alcohol entirely or limit its use to occasional small amounts. Alcohol is a simple sugar, rapidly absorbed by the body. Like other sugars, alcohol increases hypoglycemia symptoms; excessive use can increase anxiety and mood swings. (See the preceding section on sugar for a thorough discussion of this process.) This can be particularly pronounced in women with PMS-related hypoglycemia.

Once alcohol has been absorbed and assimilated, it is primarily metabolized by the liver. This is a complex process requiring much work on the part of the body. Excessive intake of alcohol can overwhelm the liver's ability to process it, leading to toxic by-products that can themselves affect mood. Too much alcohol can also impede the body's ability to detoxify other chemicals—including drugs, hormones such as estrogen, and pesticides—that we take into our bodies by choice or through environmental contact. As a result, toxic levels of these chemicals can build up in the body, worsening anxiety.

Excessive levels of estrogen seen in women with PMS, young women on birth control pills, and menopausal women on estrogen replacement therapy have been linked to altered mood states and anxiety. This can occur when the therapeutic estrogen dose prescribed by the physician is in excess of the body's needs and the body cannot detoxify it efficiently through healthy liver metabolism.

Alcohol, an irritant to the liver as well as to other parts of the digestive tract, may be used by the body for immediate energy or stored in the liver or in the rest of the body as fat. Unfortunately, the liver cannot convert alcohol to a storage form of glucose. As a result, the amount of fat stored in the liver can increase with excessive alcohol use. Alcohol raises the liver enzyme level, leading to liver inflammation (or hepatitis). Eventually the chemical by-products of alcohol and the fat derived from alcohol can cause scarring and shrinkage of the liver, leading to functional impairment of the liver and cirrhosis.

In addition, alcohol irritates the lining of the upper digestive tract, including the esophagus, stomach, and upper part of the small intestine. It also causes irritation and inflammation of the pancreas. Over time, this can result in worsening of hypoglycemia and diabetes as well as impaired absorption and assimilation of essential nutrients from the small intestine. Certain of these nutrients, such as the B vitamins, are necessary to stabilize these conditions.

The nervous system is particularly susceptible to the deleterious effects of alcohol, which readily crosses the blood-brain barrier and destroys brain cells. Alcohol can cause profound behavioral and psychological changes in women who use it excessively. Symptoms include emotional upset, irrational anger, emotional outbursts, dizziness, poor judgment, loss of memory, mental impairment, poor coordination, and difficulty in walking.

Symptoms of emotional upset triggered by alcohol can also be caused by candida overgrowth, since candida thrives on the sugar in alcohol. Alcohol can thus promote a tendency toward chronic candida infections. Women with candida-related mood upset and fatigue need to avoid alcohol entirely. Furthermore, many women with allergies are sensitive to the yeast in alcohol, which worsens their allergic symptoms.

Given the preceding information on alcohol's adverse effects, I recommend that women with anxiety symptoms use alcohol only very rarely. When used carefully—not exceeding 4 ounces of wine per day, 12 ounces of beer, or 1 ounce of hard liquor—alcohol can have a delightfully relaxing effect in women who have normal energy levels. It can make us more sociable and enhance the taste of food.

However, women who are particularly susceptible to the negative effects of alcohol shouldn't drink at all. If you entertain a great deal and enjoy social drinking, try nonalcoholic beverages. A nonalcoholic cocktail, such as mineral water with a twist of lime or lemon or a dash of bitters, is a good substitute. "Near beer" is a nonalcoholic beer substitute that tastes quite good. Light wine and beer have a lower alcohol content than hard liquor, liqueurs, and regular wine.

## Food Additives

Several thousand chemical additives are currently used in commercial food manufacturing. Some of the most popular, including aspartame (NutraSweet™), monosodium glutamate (MSG), nitrates, and nitrites, produce allergic and anxiety-like symptoms in many people. I have had patients complain that the use of the artificial sweetener aspartame precipitated panic-like symptoms, such as rapid heartbeat, shallow breathing, headaches, anxiety, spaciness, and dizziness. Since aspartame is used in so many processed diet foods, susceptible women may need to avoid low-calorie, sugar-free drinks, jams, desserts, and other foods. If you are susceptible to aspartame, be sure to carefully read the labels of any processed diet foods before you buy them.

Many women are very susceptible to the chemical MSG, a flavor enhancer that is often used in food preparation in Chinese restaurants. MSG causes headaches and anxiety episodes in some people, and patients have also reported that this chemical increased their food cravings and food addictions. If you are sensitive to MSG, check labels of bottled dressing and sauces to make sure that it is not an ingredient. Also, eat at Chinese restaurants that advertise "No MSG." Many restaurants are aware of the common sensitivity to MSG and forgo using it in their food preparation.

Nitrates and nitrites can produce allergies also. These chemicals are used as preservatives in many foods, especially cured meats such as hot dogs, bacon, and ham. Be sure to check the labels on foods that you suspect might contain nitrates or nitrites if you are sensitive to these chemicals.

## Wheat and Other Gluten-Containing Grains

Women who have brain chemistry imbalances, food allergies, stress-related digestive problems like irritable bowel syndrome, PMS or menopause-related mood problems may have difficulty tolerating wheat. The protein in wheat, called gluten, is highly allergenic and difficult for the body to break down, absorb, and assimilate. Women with wheat intolerance are prone to mood imbalances, fatigue, depression, bloating, intestinal gas and bowel changes.

In my clinical experience, wheat consumption can worsen emotional symptoms and fatigue if you are nutritionally sensitive and also suffering from anxiety or depression. I have also seen this occur with my PMS patients during the week or two before the onset of menses. Many menopausal women tolerate wheat poorly because their digestive tracts are beginning to show the wear and tear of aging and they don't produce enough enzymes to handle wheat easily.

Women with allergies often find that wheat intensifies nasal and sinus congestion as well as fatigue. I also find that women with poor resistance and a tendency toward infections may need to eliminate wheat in order to boost their immune function. Because wheat is leavened with yeast, it should be also avoided by women with candida infections.

If you are suffering from anxiety, panic attacks and sensitivity to stress, you should probably eliminate wheat from your diet. Oats and rye, which also contain gluten, should be eliminated along with wheat. (Gluten-free oats, however, are available in health food stores like Whole Foods Market.) Many allergic and anxious, stressed and fatigued women may find that they don't handle corn well, either, and should only use it in small amounts since it can adversely affect your brain chemistry.

Happily, there are many great and delicious alternatives once you embark on a gluten-free diet. These include grains such as brown rice, millet, quinoa, buckwheat and amaranth. I have found over the years that the least stressful grain for severely stressed women is buckwheat, probably because it is not commonly eaten in our society. Another factor could be that it is not in the same plant family as wheat and other grains. Other less frequently used grains such as and amaranth may be tried as well. These are the grain base of many pastas and cereals available in health food stores. Delicious gluten-free breads, crackers, pasta, cookies, cakes and flours for baking are all readily available in health food stores, many supermarkets and on the Internet.

Even non-grain flours such as nut flours made from almonds and hazelnuts as well as garbanzo bean flour can be used to make scrumptious low-carbohydrate baked goods. This is a great option if you need to follow a low-carbohydrate, high protein diet for relief of your anxiety and stress symptoms.

## Salt

While salt is essential for our health, some research studies suggest that a high salt intake in the diet can actually increase anxiety and panic attacks. While the research results of different studies are mixed, you should watch your salt intake carefully and avoid excessive intake for optimal health and well-being.

Too much salt in the diet can cause many physical problems. It can trigger bloating and fluid retention seen in PMS and menopause which are also commonly linked to mood imbalances. It worsens high blood pressure, and is a risk factor in the development of osteoporosis in menopausal women. In addition, salt can deplete the body of potassium, a mineral necessary for healthy nervous system function, energy and stamina.

Unfortunately, most processed foods contain large amounts of salt. Frozen and canned foods are often loaded with salt. In fact, one frozen-food entree can contribute as much as one-half teaspoon of salt to your daily intake. Large amounts of salt are also commonly found in the American diet as table salt (sodium chloride), MSG (monosodium glutamate) and a variety of food additives. Fast foods such as hamburgers, hot dogs, french fries, pizza, and tacos are full of salt and saturated fats. Common processed foods such as soups, potato chips, cheese, olives, salad dressings, and ketchup (to name only a few) are also very high in salt. To make matters worse, many people use too much salt while cooking and seasoning their meals.

For women of all ages, I recommend eliminating added salt in your meals. For flavor, use seasonings such as garlic, herbs, spices, and lemon juice. Avoid processed foods that are high in salt, including canned foods, olives, pickles, potato chips, tortilla chips, ketchup, and salad dressings. Learn to read labels and look for the word sodium (salt). If it appears high on the list of ingredients, don't buy the product. Many items in health food stores are labeled "no salt added." Some supermarkets offer "no added salt" foods in their diet or health food sections.

## Summary Chart: Foods to Avoid

Coffee
Tea (containing caffeine)
Chocolate
Dairy products
Salt
Soft drinks containing caffeine
Sugar
Alcohol
Foods and beverages flavored with aspartame (NutraSweet™)
Foods and beverages flavored with monosodium glutamate (MSG)
Wheat and other gluten-containing grains

## Foods that Help Relieve Anxiety

The foods you should eat when anxious, depressed, or fatigued should leave you feeling as good as, or better than, you felt before the meal. These foods should also support and accelerate the healing process of the illness that underlies the emotional symptoms. To achieve these goals means initially limiting your diet to low-stress foods. As your anxiety symptoms diminish, you can eat a wider range of foods. Begin to develop an awareness of how your food selections affect your emotional well-being. If a particular food makes you feel anxious, jittery, depressed, or fatigued when you eat it, you should eliminate it.

I have found that certain groups of foods are tolerated by nearly everyone, even women who are anxious and upset. These foods include most vegetables, fruits, starches, grains such as brown rice, millet, buckwheat, quinoa and amaranth and corn (in women who do not have severe PMS or food allergies), nuts, seeds, fish, free-range poultry and monounsaturated oils like olive oil and almond oil. These should be your core food selection.

In this section I describe the anti-anxiety and mood-stabilizing effects of these beneficial foods.

### Vegetables

These are outstanding foods for the relief of stress. Many vegetables are high in calcium, magnesium, and potassium—important minerals that help improve stamina, endurance, and vitality. Both magnesium and potassium, used in supplemental form in clinical studies, have been shown to reduce depression and increase energy levels dramatically.

For women who suffer from tension and anxiety, the essential minerals in vegetables have a relaxant effect, relieving muscular tension and calming the emotions. Both calcium and magnesium act as natural tranquilizers, a real benefit for women suffering from stress and upset. The potassium content of vegetables helps relieve congestive symptoms by reducing fluid retention and bloating. Some of the best sources for these minerals include Swiss chard, spinach, broccoli, beet greens, mustard greens, and kale.

Many vegetables are high in vitamin C, which helps strengthen capillaries, thereby facilitating the flow of essential nutrients throughout the body, as well as the flow of waste products out. Vitamin C is also an important anti-stress vitamin because it promotes healthy adrenal hormone production (the adrenal glands help us deal with stress). This is particularly important for women with anxiety caused by emotional upset, allergies, or stress from other origins, such as the environment.

Vitamin C is also important for immune function and wound healing. Its anti-infectious properties may help reduce the tendency towards respiratory, bladder, and vaginal infections. Vegetables high in vitamin C include Brussels sprouts, broccoli, cauliflower, kale, peppers, parsley, peas, tomatoes, and potatoes.

Carrots, spinach, squash, turnip greens, collards, parsley, green onions, and kale are among the vegetables highest in vitamin A. Vitamin A strengthens the cell walls and protects the mucous membranes. This helps protect you from respiratory disease as well as allergic episodes. Vitamin A is important for women with anxiety whose resistance is low and who are thus prone to allergies and infections. Vitamin A deficiency has been linked to fatigue as well as night blindness, skin aging, loss of smell, loss of appetite, and softening of bones and teeth. Luckily, it is easy to get an abundance of vitamin A from vegetables.

Vegetables are composed primarily of water and carbohydrates. They tend to be easy to digest because they contain very little protein and fat. However, some women find that they have fewer digestive problems with cooked vegetables. Cooking breaks down and softens the fiber in the vegetables, making less work for the body in the digestion process. Steaming is the best cooking method, because it preserves the essential nutrients. Some women with extreme stress and fatigue may even want to puree their vegetables in a blender. As you begin to recover your emotional balance and energy level, I recommend adding raw foods such as salads, vegetable juices, and raw vegetables to your meals for more texture and variety.

## Fruits

Fruits also contain a wide range of nutrients that can relieve anxiety and stress. Like many vegetables, fruits are an excellent source of vitamin C, which is important for healthy blood vessels and blood circulation, as well as for anti-stress and immune-stimulant properties. Almost all fruits contain some vitamin C, the best sources being berries and melons. These fruits are also good sources of bioflavonoids, another essential nutrient that affects blood vessel strength and permeability as well as your hormonal balance. Vitamin C and bioflavonoids are an excellent combination for women who suffer from anxiety and mood swings due to hormone related conditions like PMS and menopause.

Bioflavonoids also have an anti-inflammatory effect, important to women with allergies, menstrual cramps, or arthritis. Bioflavonoids are supportive of the female reproductive tract and can improve mood and increase energy levels. Although citrus fruits (oranges, grapefruits) are excellent sources of bioflavonoids and vitamin C, they are highly acidic and difficult for many women with food allergies or sensitive digestive tracts to digest; therefore, such women should avoid them in the early stages of treatment.

Certain fruits — including raisins, blackberries, and bananas — are excellent sources of calcium and magnesium, two essential minerals for healthy nervous system and muscular function. Raisins and bananas are also exceptional sources of potassium, good for women with excessive fatigue and bloating. All fruits, in fact, are excellent sources of potassium that helps to support your energy and vitality that can be depleted if you are chronically overly stressed and anxious.

Eat fruits whole to benefit from their high fiber content, which helps to prevent constipation and other digestive irregularities that are often stress related. For snacks and desserts, fresh fruits are excellent substitutes for anxiety-worsening, high sugar content cookies, candies, cakes, and other foods high in refined sugar. Although fruit is high in sugar, its high fiber content helps slow down absorption of the sugar into the blood circulation and thereby helps stabilize the blood sugar level.

I recommend, however, that women with anxiety and stress do not consume fruit juices. Fruit juice does not contain the bulk or fiber of the whole fruit. As a result, it acts more like table sugar and can destabilize your blood sugar level dramatically when used to excess. This can exacerbate anxiety, jitteriness, shakiness, fatigue and mood swings.

## Starches

Potatoes, sweet potatoes, and yams are soft, well-tolerated carbohydrates that also provide fiber and small amounts of easy-to-digest protein for women with anxiety and nervous tension. Like the other complex carbohydrates, starches calm the mood by helping to regulate the blood sugar level. You can steam, mash, bake, and eat them alone, or include them in other low-stress dishes and casseroles. Starches combine very well with a variety of vegetables and can form the basis of delicious, low-stress meals. You can also combine them with lentils or split peas in soup.

Potatoes, especially sweet potatoes, are an exceptional source of vitamin A, so they can help boost resistance to infections and allergies. Potatoes and yams are also good sources of vitamin C and several of the B vitamins that help women handle anxiety and stress better and reduce fatigue.

## Legumes

Beans and peas are excellent sources of calcium, magnesium, and potassium, which are necessary for healthy nervous system function, as well as for their emotional and muscle-relaxant properties. I highly recommend their use in a diet to combat depression and fatigue. Legumes are also very high in vitamin B-complex and vitamin B6, necessary nutrients for the relief and prevention of anxiety, menstrual fatigue, PMS symptoms, and cramps. They are also excellent sources of protein and, when eaten with grains, provide all the essential amino acids. Good examples of low-stress grain and legume combinations include meals of beans and buckwheat, or corn bread and split pea soup.

Legumes provide an excellent, easily utilized source of protein and can be substituted for meat at many meals. Legumes are an excellent source of fiber that can help normalize bowel function. They digest slowly and can help to regulate the blood sugar level, a trait they share with whole grains. As a result, legumes are an ideal food for women with blood sugar imbalances caused by diabetes, anxiety, nervous tension, and diet.

Some women find gas to be a problem when they eat beans. You can minimize gas by taking digestive enzymes and eating beans in small quantities. Also, because legumes contain high levels of protein, women with severe fatigue or digestive problems may find them difficult to digest at first. For easier digestibility, I recommend beginning with green beans, green peas, split peas, lentils, lima beans, fresh sprouts, and possibly tofu (if you handle soy products well). As your energy level improves, add delicious legumes such as black beans, pinto beans, kidney beans, and chickpeas. These foods are high in iron and tend to be good sources of copper and zinc.

## Whole Grains

Although you should eliminate some grains from your diet (especially wheat and other gluten-containing grains) when first starting an anti-anxiety program, many whole grains have tremendous health benefits for women suffering from nervous tension. Whole grains are excellent sources of mood-stabilizing nutrients like vitamin B-complex, vitamin E, many essential minerals, complex carbohydrates, protein, essential fatty acids, and fiber. Like legumes, whole grains help stabilize blood sugar levels to prevent hypoglycemia-triggered anxiety symptoms.

Brown rice, quinoa and millet are good choices for women with mild to moderate anxiety symptoms, as are buckwheat and more exotic grain alternatives, such as amaranth. Pasta, cereals, flour, and other foods made from these grain alternatives can be purchased in health food stores, many supermarkets and on the Internet. For baking, non-grain flours such as almond flour and garbanzo bean flour are great low-carbohydrate alternatives.

Women with allergy-related anxiety symptoms need to be careful not to overeat any one grain. Rotating a variety of gluten-free grains in the diet can prevent anxiety caused by allergic reactions or fatigue. Besides eating corn and rice as primary grains, you can find pasta and noodles, as well as flour for baking, made from these grains. Use rice and corn tortillas instead of those made of wheat.

## Seeds and Nuts

Seeds and nuts are the best sources of the two essential fatty acids, linoleic acid and alpha-linolenic acid. These fatty acids provide the raw materials your body needs to produce the beneficial prostaglandin hormones. Adequate levels of essential fatty acids in your diet are very important in preventing both the emotional and physical symptoms of PMS, menopause, emotional upsets, and allergies. The best sources of both fatty acids are raw flax, chia and hemp seeds. Other seeds, such as sesame and sunflower seeds, are excellent sources of linoleic acid.

Seeds and nuts are also good sources of the B-complex vitamins and vitamin E, both of which are important anti-stress factors for women with muscle tension and emotional stress symptoms. These nutrients also help regulate hormonal balance. Like vegetables, seeds and nuts are very high in the essential minerals such as magnesium, calcium, and potassium needed by women with excessive muscle tension and emotional stress symptoms. Particularly beneficial are sesame seeds, sunflower seeds, pistachios, pecans, and almonds.

Nuts and seeds are very high in calories and can be difficult to digest, especially if they are roasted and salted. Therefore, you should eat them only in small to moderate amounts. Flaxseed oil is one of the best sources of the essential fatty acids needed for production of the beneficial prostaglandin hormones. It has a rich, golden color and may be used as a butter substitute on vegetables, rice, potatoes, pasta, and popcorn. Unlike butter, flax oil cannot be used for cooking. Cook foods first; then add flax oil to the food for flavoring just before serving.

The oils in all seeds and nuts are very perishable, so avoid exposing them to light, heat, and oxygen. Refrigerate all shelled seeds and nuts as well as their oils to prevent rancidity. Try to eat them raw, and shell them yourself. This gives you the benefit of their essential fatty acids, and you'll also avoid the negative effects of too much salt. Seeds and nuts make a wonderful garnish on salads, vegetable dishes, and casseroles.

## Poultry and Fish

I generally recommend eating red meat in moderation. Meats such as beef, pork, and lamb contain saturated fats and hard to digest protein. They should be eaten only occasionally, and I recommend purchasing grass fed, organic red meats that are lower in fat.

If you do want to eat a meat-based diet, your best choice is fish or free range poultry and eggs. Unlike other meat, fish contains omega-3 fatty acid that can help to relax your mood as well as your tense muscles. Fish is an excellent source of minerals, especially iodine and potassium. Particularly good selections for women with anxiety are salmon, tuna, mackerel, halibut and trout. Free range poultry and fertile eggs are also good choices for women who feel better on a higher protein diet.

In general, most Americans eat much more protein than is necessary to be healthy. Excessive amounts of protein are difficult to digest and stress the kidneys. If you do include meat in your anxiety program, use it in moderate amounts (6 ounces or less of meat per day). Instead of using meat as your only source of protein, increase your intake of grains, beans, raw seeds, and nuts, which contain not only protein but also many other important anti-anxiety nutrients.

I also suggest buying meat from organic, free range animals, because their exposure to pesticides, antibiotics, and hormones has been reduced. If you find meat difficult to digest, you may be deficient in hydrochloric acid and digestive enzymes like pancreatin, bromelain and papain. Try taking these in supplement form with any meal containing meat to see if your digestion improves.

## Substitute Healthy Ingredients in Recipes

In this section, I want to provide you with more detailed information on how to substitute healthy ingredients in recipes or making substitutions for high-stress foods that you've currently been eating. Learning how to make substitutions for high-stress ingredients in familiar recipes allows you to prepare your favorite foods without compromising your emotional or physical health.

Many recipes contain ingredients that women with anxiety and stress should avoid, particularly the high stress foods such as caffeine, alcohol, sugar, chocolate, and dairy products. By replacing these with healthier ingredients, you can continue to make many recipes that appeal to you. I have recommended this approach for years to my patients, who are pleased to find that they can still have their favorite dishes, but in much healthier versions.

Some women choose to totally eliminate high stress ingredients from a recipe. For example, you can make pasta with tomato sauce but eliminate the Parmesan cheese topping and use gluten-free pasta. Greek salad can be made without the feta cheese or with just a sprinkling of sheep or goat feta cheese that is often better tolerated than cheese and other dairy products made from cow's milk.

Some of my patients even make pizza with vegan cheese or without cheese, layering tomato sauce and lots of vegetables on the crust and adding delicious herbs or flavoring. In many cases, the high-stress ingredients are not necessary to make foods taste good. Always remember, they can worsen your anxiety symptoms and impair your health.

If you want to use a particular high stress ingredient, you can usually substantially reduce the amount of that ingredient you use, while still retaining the flavor and taste. Most of us have palates jaded by too much fat, salt, sugar, and other flavorings. In many dishes, we taste only the additives; we never really enjoy the delicious flavors of the foods themselves. Now that I regularly substitute low-stress ingredients in my cooking, I enjoy the subtle taste of the dishes much more. Also, my health and vitality continue to improve with the deletion of high stress ingredients. The following information tells you how to substitute healthy ingredients in your own recipes or for your high stress favorite foods. The substitutions are simple to make and should benefit your health greatly.

## Substitutions for Caffeinated Foods and Beverages

*Drink substitutes for coffee and black tea.* The best substitutes are the grain-based coffee beverages, such as Postum and Cafix. Some women may find the abrupt discontinuance of coffee too difficult because of withdrawal symptoms, such as headaches. If this concerns you, decrease your total coffee intake gradually to only one or one-half cup per day and use grain-based substitutes for your other cups. This will help prevent withdrawal symptoms.

*Drink decaffeinated coffee or tea during transition.* If you cannot give up coffee, start by substituting water-processed decaffeinated coffee for the real thing. Then try to wean yourself from coffee altogether, or use a coffee substitute.

*Use herbal teas for energy and vitality.* Many women with anxiety and excessive stress mistakenly drink coffee as a pick-me-up to be able to function during the day. Use peppermint or ginger teas instead. These teas are energizing but won't have a negative effect on your mood. If you can handle a small amount of caffeine, then green tea is a great option. It has a slight stimulant effect as well as many other health benefits. To make ginger tea, grate a few teaspoons of fresh ginger root into a pot of hot water; boil and steep.

*Substitute carob for chocolate.* Unsweetened carob tastes like chocolate but doesn't contain the caffeine found in chocolate. It is also naturally sweeter than chocolate, which is bitter and requires a lot of anxiety-worsening sugar to improve the taste. A member of the legume family, carob is high in calcium. You can purchase it in chunk form as a substitute for chocolate candy or as a powder for use in baking or drinks. Be careful, however, not to overindulge; carob, like chocolate, is high in calories and fat. Consider it a treat and a cooking aid for use in small amounts only.

## Substitutions for Sugar

Many women are addicted to sugar, which can worsen anxiety symptoms. Most of us grew up on highly sugared soft drinks, candy, and rich pastries—no wonder the incidence of diabetes is soaring among our population. I have found that as women decrease their sugar intake, most begin to really enjoy the subtle flavors of the foods they eat. There are a number of great sugar substitutes on the market that won't worsen your mood symptoms and several even have health benefits. These include:

*Substitute healthy sweetening agents.* Stevia and xylitol are two of my favorites. Stevia is an herbal sweetener that is calorie free. Thus, it is helpful if you are on a weight loss program or don't want the extra calories found in other sweeteners such as sugar or honey. Because stevia contains no calories from sugar, it does not create imbalances in the blood sugar level. This is very beneficial if you suffer from hypoglycemia or diabetes.

Xylitol is a wonderful sweetener that is derived from woody fibrous plant material. It gives a delicious flavor to baked goods, desserts and beverages without the health problems related to table sugar like diabetes, candida infections, obesity and tooth decay. Even better, xylitol is as sweet as sugar but has only two thirds the calories.

Xylitol is absorbed more slowly than sugar so is helpful for diabetes, has antibacterial and antifungal properties and helps promote healthy teeth and gums. It is also found naturally in guavas, pears, blackberries, raspberries, aloe vera, eggplant, peas, green beans and corn.

*Substitute concentrated sweeteners.* Concentrated sweeteners such as honey and maple syrup have a sweeter taste per quantity used than table sugar. Using these substitutes will enable you to cut down on the amount of sugar used. If you use a concentrated sweetener in place of sugar in an ordinary recipe, reduce the liquid content in the recipe by one-fourth cup. If no liquid is used in the recipe, add 3 to 5 tablespoons of flour for each three-fourths cup of concentrated sweetener.

*Substitute fruit for sugar in pastries.* In making muffins and cookies, you may want to try removing sugar altogether and adding extra fruits and nuts. Many of my patients like to use applesauce and bananas as sweeteners in baked goods to cut down the need for sugar.

## Substitutions for Alcohol

*Use low-alcohol or nonalcoholic products for drinking or cooking.* There are many delicious low-alcohol and nonalcoholic wines and beers for sale in supermarkets and liquor stores. Many of these taste quite good and can be used for meals or at social occasions. In addition, you can substitute low-alcohol or nonalcoholic wine or beer when cooking or preparing sauces and marinades. You will retain much of the flavor that alcohol imparts, and you'll decrease the stress factor substantially.

*Use sparkling water for parties and social events.* Many of us enjoy holding a beverage while socializing. Instead of alcoholic beverages like wine, hard liquor or a mixed drink, consider sparkling water with a twist of lemon or lime. A splash of bitters is also excellent. Or, combine sparkling water with a little fruit juice for a festive drink.

## Substitutions for Dairy Products

*Eliminate or decrease the amount of cheese you use in food preparation and cooking.* If you must use cheese in cooking, decrease the amount in the recipe by three-fourths so that it becomes a flavoring or garnish rather than a major source of fat and protein. For example, use two teaspoons of Parmesan cheese on top of a casserole instead of one-half cup.

*Use vegan, soy or rice cheese without casein in food preparation and cooking.* These nondairy cheeses are all excellent substitutes for cheese. They are all lower in fat and salt, and the fat it does contain isn't saturated. Health food stores offer many brands that come in different flavors, such as mozzarella, cheddar, American, and jack. The quality of these products keeps improving all the time.

You can use soy, vegan and rice cheeses in sandwiches, salads, pizzas, lasagnas, and casseroles. You can also use small amount of goat or sheep cheese in recipes as they tend to be more digestible and better tolerated than cheeses and other dairy products.

In some recipes you can replace cheese with soft tofu. I have done this often with lasagna, layering the lasagna noodles with tofu and topping with melted soy cheese for a delicious dish. The tofu, which is bland, takes on the taste of the tomato sauce.

*Replace milk and yogurt in recipes.* For milk, substitute rice, coconut, almond, hempseed, flaxseed, sunflower seed, grain and soymilk. All of these milks come in various flavors including unsweetened, vanilla, strawberry, chocolate and carob. Three to four glasses of soymilk each day provides a significant amount of the soy isoflavones, which are estrogen-like chemicals that help to regulate mood during the perimenopausal and menopausal years. Soy also helps to regulate cholesterol levels in middle-aged women. Many nondairy milks are good sources of calcium and can be used for drinking, eating, or baking. Soy and nut milks are available at most health food stores.

For yogurt, substitute almond, coconut and soy yogurt. Several excellent brands of non-dairy yogurt are available in health food stores in plain, vanilla, and fruit flavors. The taste is excellent and approximates that of yogurt. They are good substitutes for both cooking and baking.

*Substitute flaxseed oil for butter.* Flaxseed oil is the best substitute for butter I have found. It is a rich, golden oil that looks and tastes quite a bit like butter. It is delicious on anything you would normally top with butter—toast, rice, popcorn, steamed vegetables, or potatoes. Flaxseed oil is extremely high in beneficial omega-3 essential fatty acids—the type of fat that is very healthy for a woman's body, as well as promotes a balanced mood and brain chemistry. Essential fatty acids also improve vitality, enhance circulation, and help promote healthy hormonal function.

Flaxseed oil is quite perishable, however, because it is sensitive to heat and light. You can't cook with it—cook the food first and add the flaxseed oil before serving. Also, be sure to keep it refrigerated. Flaxseed oil has so many health benefits that I highly recommend its use. You can find it in most health food stores.

## Substitutions for Red Meat

*Substitute turkey, chicken, eggs, beans, tofu, or seeds in recipes.* You can often modify recipes calling for red meat by substituting ground turkey, ground chicken, or tofu. For example, use ground turkey or crumble up tofu to simulate the texture of hamburger and add to recipes like enchiladas, tacos, chili, meatloaf, and ground beef casseroles. Ground turkey and ground chicken are very flavorful. The tofu takes on the flavor of the sauce used in the dish and is indistinguishable from red meat. I often do this when cooking at home.

In addition, many substitute meat products are available in health food stores. These products include tofu hot dogs, hamburgers, bacon, ham, chicken, and turkey. The variety is astounding, and many of these meat substitutes taste remarkably good. The quality of these products has dramatically improved over the years. However, if you are allergic to soy, you should avoid these substitutes and use organic, free range chicken and turkey sausages and hot dogs, free range organic beef or bison hamburgers and other healthier types of meat, instead.

When making salads that call for ham or bacon, such as chef's salad or Cobb salad, substitute turkey bacon and add kidney beans, garbanzo beans, hard boiled eggs, or sunflower seeds. These will provide the needed protein, yet be more healthful and, often, more easily digestible. You can also sprinkle sunflower seeds on top of casseroles for extra protein and essential fatty acids. When making stir-fries; substitute turkey, chicken, tofu, almonds, or sprouts for red meat.

## Substitutions for Wheat and Gluten-Containing Grains

*Use whole grain non-wheat flour.* Substitute whole grain non-wheat flours, such as rice or quinoa flour. These whole grain flours are good sources of essential nutrients, including vitamin B-complex and many minerals. They are also higher in fiber content. These nutrients help to correct estrogen dominance and promote hormonal balance. Unlike the gluten-containing grains like wheat, rye and oats, they do not promote mood related symptoms. Rice flour makes excellent cookies, cakes, and other pastries.

You can also use nut flour and garbanzo bean flour if you want to avoid the use of grain based flours altogether. These flours can be used to make the most scrumptious and tasty low carbohydrate breads, pancakes, cakes, cookies and tarts. I especially love using nut flour for my delicious and healthy non-gluten, dairy free baked goods.

When purchasing flour based products, you can readily find breads, crackers, cookies, cakes, pasta and cereals made from then gluten-free grains, nuts and beans. They are available in health food stores, many supermarkets and on the Internet.

## Substitutions for Salt

*Substitute potassium-based products for table salt (sodium chloride).* Potassium-based products, such as Morton's Salt Substitute, are much healthier and will not aggravate heart disease or hypertension.

*Use powdered seaweeds* such as kelp or nori to season vegetables, grains, and salads. They are high in essential iodine and trace elements.

*Use herbs instead of salt for flavoring.* Their flavors are much more subtle and will help even the most jaded palate appreciate the taste of fresh fruits, vegetables, and meats.

*Use liquid flavoring agents with advertised low-sodium content.* Low-sodium soy sauce and Bragg's Amino Acids, a liquid soybean-based flavoring agent, are delicious when used as salt substitutes in cooking. Add them to soups, casseroles, stir-fries, and other dishes at the end of the cooking process. You need only a small amount for intense flavoring.

**Substitutes for Common High-Stress Ingredients**

| High-Stress Ingredient | Low-Stress Substitute |
| --- | --- |
| ¾ cup sugar | ¾ cup xylitol<br>½ cup honey<br>¼ cup molasses<br>½ cup maple syrup<br>½ ounce barley malt<br>1 cup apple butter<br>2 cups apple juice |
| 1 cup milk | 1 cup soy, rice, nut, or grain milk |
| 1 cup yogurt | 1 cup soy, rice, or other nondairy yogurt |
| 1 tablespoon butter | 1 tablespoon flax oil (must be used raw and unheated) |
| ½ teaspoon salt | 1 tablespoon miso<br>½ teaspoon potassium chloride salt substitute<br>½ teaspoon Mrs. Dash, Spike<br>½ teaspoon herbs (basil, tarragon, oregano, etc.) |
| 1 ½ cups cocoa | 1 cup powdered carob |
| 1 square chocolate | ¾ tablespoon powdered carob |
| 1 tablespoon coffee | 1 tablespoon decaffeinated coffee<br>1 tablespoon Postum, Cafix, or other grain-based coffee substitute |
| 4 ounces wine | 4 ounces light wine |
| 8 ounces beer | 8 ounces near beer |
| 1 cup white flour | 1 to 1 ¼ cup rice, quinoa, nut or garbanzo or other bean flour. |

# 6

## Menus, Meal Plans & Recipes

Enjoying a delicious meal is one of life's great pleasures. Few things compare to spending a relaxed evening with our friends and family, dining on a scrumptious meal prepared with love and care. It is also a delightful treat to savor new flavors and tastes. The good news is that a diet that supports a healthy mood and balanced brain chemistry can be just as delicious as your current food habits!

In this chapter, I share with you meal plans and recipes that I have created that not only taste delicious but are filled with essential nutrients that will help to relieve and prevent symptoms of anxiety, panic attacks and stress. These meal plans will help you create a foundation of healthful eating that will support your brain and nervous system chemistry, your hormones, immunity and health in general.

Food has a powerful effect on our mood. I have seen with many of my patients that they were unknowingly eating foods that were contributing to their mood-related symptoms. For example, many of my patients were eating foods with too much sugar or caffeine that can worsen anxiety and even trigger panic attacks. Sugar and caffeine also trigger moodiness, anxiety and irritability in women who are struggling with PMS and menopause. Some of my patients have had undiagnosed food allergies or intolerances to common foods like milk products and wheat that were worsening their mood and stress symptoms.

In addition, food fills emotional as well as nutritional needs for many women. For example, women commonly snack on "junk foods" like cookies, colas, candy bars, and other high-stress foods when they are feeling anxious. While these foods give an immediate emotional boost, the ingredients and additives contained in them often make the anxiety symptoms worse over time.

These are just a few examples of how food can affect your reactions to stressful situations and set off anxiety and panic attacks. One of my patients, Lauren, is so sensitive to caffeine that if she even drinks a low caffeine content beverage like green tea, she will have a full-fledged anxiety episode with shakiness, chest tightness and insomnia. Green tea is a very healthful beverage for most women with many benefits but not for Lauren who cannot handle even the small amount of caffeine found in green tea!

It is very important to be aware of your specific sensitivities and intolerances to foods when trying to eliminate anxiety and panic attacks. I have found with my own patients that once they are aware of the beneficial role that proper food selection can play in preventing and relieving anxiety and stress, they were always motivated to shift their eating habits toward more healthy choices. Most of my patients really enjoyed exploring new, more healthful foods. Best of all, the benefits of choosing foods that stabilized their mood were often apparent quickly, especially when combined with a therapeutic nutritional supplement program.

Making the transition, however, may present some challenges. Many of us tend to be creatures of habit, so the prospect of changing our food selection may sometimes appear difficult and intimidating. Over the years, my patients did best when I provided specific guidelines to help them through the transition period.

When changing from a high-stress diet to an anxiety relief food plan, my patients requested specific menus and meal plans. Although information on which foods to eat and which to avoid is tremendously helpful, most women want to know how to take the next step and combine the right foods in healthful meals. Many of my patients benefited enormously from these simple and easy-to-follow guidelines, so I have included the information in this chapter for your benefit, too

Unfortunately, most cookbooks do not adequately address a woman's needs for specific nutrients when they are suffering from anxiety, stress and panic attacks. Many contain recipes that are too high in the nutrients that can worsen mood imbalances such as sugar, caffeine, alcohol, chocolate, animal fats, dairy products and too much salt.

Many nutrition-conscious cookbooks present low-calorie "light dishes" that eliminate the high-stress ingredients, but still don't give women suffering from anxiety and stress symptoms the therapeutic levels of specific nutrients they need.

To help with this issue, I have also created a number of recipes that I have included in this chapter to further support your transition towards restoring a healthy and balanced mood. My patients have found this extremely beneficial and have given me very positive feedback about their enjoyment of many of these dishes as well as receiving therapeutic results. My own friends and family have also greatly enjoyed these healthy dishes and meals over the years.

I have found that no one diet fits the needs of all different body types. Because of this I have included menus and delicious recipes for women who prefer a vegetarian emphasis, high complex carbohydrate diet as well as dishes and entrees for women who feel their best on a high protein meat-based diet. All of these meal plans and recipes contain ingredients most suitable for providing relief for women with anxiety and stress symptoms. In addition, the high stress ingredients that can worsen your symptoms have been eliminated.

Because many women lead busy lives and have many demands on their time, I've devised recipes that are quick and easy to prepare. I have found that anything too complicated doesn't work for many of my patients. Best of all, these recipes are delicious as well as healthful. I hope that you find trying these new dishes to be a delightful adventure as well.

Before discussing the actual meals plans, and recipes, I want to emphasize three principles that will make the transition process easier for you.

### Make All Dietary Changes Gradually

Make the transition to a healthful anxiety relief diet in an easy and non-stressful manner. Don't try to change all your dietary habits at once by making a clean sweep of your refrigerator and pantry unless you feel comfortable doing this. If you can make an immediate switch over to new food choices, it is great but not mandatory. Some of my patients have been very comfortable with this. However, I have seen patients try to make such dramatic changes in their diet and come to my office in an absolute panic because the change was too quick and drastic.

Instead, make your dietary changes at a pace that works for you. You may want to gradually substitute healthy foods for the high-stress foods you have been eating. To do this, periodically review the lists of foods to limit and foods to emphasize. Each time you review this list, pick several foods that you are willing to eliminate and several to try. Review these lists as often as you choose, but do it on a regular basis. Every small change that you make in your diet can help.

### Keep Your Meals Simple and Easy to Prepare

Many women lead busy, active lives and don't have a lot of time to cook complicated meals. For that reason, I've kept my meal plans quick and simple to prepare, with the main emphasis on foods that are delicious and high in nutrition. For those who are used to eating quick meals at fast-food restaurants or commercial snack food that is high in fat, sugar, and food additives, these simple meals offer a much healthier alternative.

### Eat Smaller, More Frequent Meals or Snacks

Women with anxiety symptoms feel better if they eat more frequently during the day. This helps stabilize the blood sugar level and reduce the "roller coaster" emotional and energetic highs and lows typical of PMS and hypoglycemia. If you don't want to actually eat smaller, more frequent meals, at least eat a healthful snack each period between meals to avoid symptoms of anxiety and jitteriness. Excellent snacks combine complex carbohydrates, protein, and essential fatty acids. Good examples include raw sunflower seeds or almonds, rice cakes with almond butter or tuna fish spread, air-popped popcorn, and fresh fruit such as apples, pears, and bananas.

Let's now look at some sample meal plans for breakfast, lunch and dinner that should be helpful in providing support for a balanced, healthy mood.

Breakfast is actually the most important meal of the day. If breakfast foods containing complex carbohydrates, essential fatty acids, and protein are combined properly they can help to calm your mood. They do this by stabilizing the blood sugar level and providing the body with many important nutrients for healthy nervous system function. Healthful and nourishing foods will provide the energy and vitality you need to sail through your work and activities.

Unfortunately, many women skip breakfast entirely. This can worsen both the symptoms of anxiety and stress due to brain chemistry imbalances, hypoglycemia, PMS, menopause, food allergies, and the anxiety episodes in women with mitral valve prolapse.

Some women eat foods like doughnuts, sweet rolls, and coffee in hopes of getting quick energy, but these foods can instead increase nervous tension and anxiety. Others may eat hearty breakfasts full of high-stress foods— bacon, milk, toast, and butter. The high fat and salt content of these foods further stresses the body and impairs your health.

## Breakfast Menus

These breakfast menus have been developed to help reduce and prevent symptoms of anxiety, stress and panic attacks. All the dishes contain high levels of the essential nutrients that women with these problems need. You can use these menus as idea generators for your own meal planning.

Breakfast has been one of the easiest meals for my patients to restructure along healthier lines. It tends to be a smaller and simpler meal. You may want to make healthful dietary changes in your breakfast first and then move on to lunch and dinner.

Flax shake with protein powder
and fresh fruit
~~~~~~~~~~~~~~~

Blueberry and spirulina smoothie
~~~~~~~~~~~~~~~

Millet cereal with raisins and
cinnamon
Nondairy yogurt
Chamomile tea
~~~~~~~~~~~~~~~

Rice and flaxseed pancakes
Banana
Vanilla nondairy milk
~~~~~~~~~~~~~~~

Gluten-free waffles with sliced
bananas
Peppermint tea

Oatmeal with raspberries
Chamomile tea
~~~~~~~~~~~~~~~

Nondairy yogurt with granola
and ground flaxseed
Peppermint tea
~~~~~~~~~~~~~~~

Scrambled eggs and turkey bacon
Ginger tea
~~~~~~~~~~~~~~~

Omelette with chicken sausage
Roasted grain beverage (coffee
substitute)
~~~~~~~~~~~~~~~

Pumpkin muffins
Almond butter
Vanilla nondairy milk

## Lunch and Dinner Menus

I have included a variety of menus you can choose from when planning your meals. You can use these menu plans, or use them as idea generators, to fit your own taste and needs. These dishes contain many nutritious and healthful ingredients for relief of anxiety and stress. Use these menus as helpful guidelines throughout the entire month. Your nutritional status on a day-by-day basis determines in part how likely you are to have symptoms of anxiety and panic attacks. These dishes should help to diminish the severity of your symptoms because they eliminate high-stress foods like sugar, caffeine, alcohol and additives.

### Soup Meals
Split pea soup
Pumpkin muffins
Fresh applesauce
~~~~~~~~~~~~~~

Chicken and wild rice soup
Cole slaw
Millet bread with flaxseed oil
~~~~~~~~~~~~~~

Vegetable soup with brown rice
Steamed kale
Baked potato with flaxseed oil
Apple slices
~~~~~~~~~~~~~~

Lentil soup
Herbed brown rice
Broccoli with lemon
~~~~~~~~~~~~~~

Tomato soup
Potato salad with low-fat mayonnaise
Celery and carrot sticks
~~~~~~~~~~~~~~

### Salad Meals
Spinach salad with turkey bacon or tofu
Corn muffins with flaxseed oil
Orange slices
~~~~~~~~~~~~~~

Beet salad with goat cheese
Rice crackers with fresh fruit preserves
~~~~~~~~~~~~~~

Romaine salad with grilled salmon
Gluten-free bread and olive oil dip
~~~~~~~~~~~~~~

Low-fat potato salad
Cole slaw
Hard boiled eggs
Melon slices
~~~~~~~~~~~~~~

Mixed Vegetable Salad with Garbanzo Beans
Baked yam with flaxseed oil and cinnamon

## Meat Meals

Poached salmon with lemon
Herbed brown rice
Steamed carrots with honey
~~~~~~~~~~~~~~

Roasted chicken with herbs
Baked potato with flaxseed oil
Broccoli with lemon
~~~~~~~~~~~~~~

Broiled trout with dill
Mixed green salad with vinaigrette
Green peas and onions
Apple slices
~~~~~~~~~~~~~~

Grilled shrimp with olive oil and
lemon
Wild rice
Steamed kale
~~~~~~~~~~~~~~

## One-Dish Vegetable Meals

Vegetarian tacos with black beans,
brown rice, avocados, tomatoes,
lettuce and low-salt salsa
~~~~~~~~~~~~~~

Stir-fry with mixed vegetables,
brown rice and tofu
Orange slices
~~~~~~~~~~~~~~

Pasta with tomato sauce, broccoli,
carrots, olive oil and garlic
Green salad with vinaigrette
~~~~~~~~~~~~~~

Hummus dip
Eggplant dip (babaganoush)
Mixed raw vegetable slices
including carrots, red bell peppers,
and radishes
~~~~~~~~~~~~~~

Brown rice and almond tabouli
Mixed olives
Melon slices
~~~~~~~~~~~~~~

## Breakfast Recipes

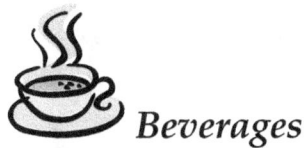 *Beverages*

These delicious drinks are made with therapeutic herbal teas, power smoothies that are rich in fruits, raw seeds, nuts, protein powder, green foods and nondairy milk that are recommended for preventing and treating your symptoms.

The ingredients contain high levels of essential nutrients that can help promote a calm and relaxing mood as well as relieve physical tension in your muscles. You can enjoy these beverages throughout the month, and not just during your symptom time, as their high mineral and other nutrient content is beneficial for the entire body.

**Relaxant Herb Tea**                                              **Serves 2**

2 cups water
1 teaspoon chamomile leaves
1 teaspoon peppermint leaves
1 teaspoon honey (if desired)

Bring the water to a boil. Place herbs in water and stir. Turn heat to low and simmer for 15 minutes.

*Peppermint and chamomile are both muscle relaxants and antispasmodic herbs, so they can provide relief of pain and cramping caused by anxiety and stress. They also help calm the mood.*

**Ginger Tea**                                                   **Serves 4**

*Ginger makes a warming, delicious tea and is beneficial to your circulation. It is also a powerful anti-inflammatory herb. If the tea is too strong add more water.*

5 cups water
3 tablespoons ginger coarsely chopped
½ lemon (optional)
Honey (or other sweetener, to taste)

Add ginger to the water in a cooking pot. Bring to a boil and then turn heat to low. Steep for 15 or 20 minutes. Squeeze lemon into tea and serve with honey or your favorite sweetener.


**Blueberry Coconut Smoothie**                                   **Serves 2**

1 cup coconut water
⅔ cup blueberries – fresh or frozen
1 heaping tablespoon raw coconut flour
1 heaping tablespoon raw almonds (10-15)
1 banana, sliced

Combine all ingredients in a blender. Puree until smooth and serve.


**Raspberry Flax Smoothie**                                      **Serves 2**

*This creamy smoothie makes a great breakfast. Flaxseed oil one is my favorite foods. It is both delicious and rich in healthy omega-3 fatty acids. It also adds extra creaminess to the smoothie.*

1 cup rice milk
⅔ cup raspberries – fresh or frozen
1 heaping tablespoon rice protein powder
1 tablespoon flaxseed oil
2 bananas, sliced

Combine all ingredients in a blender. Puree until smooth and serve.

**Delicious Green Drink**                                    **Serves 1**

½ cup Concord grape juice
¼ cup water
1 tablespoon ground flaxseed
½ teaspoon chlorella powder
½ teaspoon spirulina powder

Mix all ingredients together in a glass or puree in a blender.

**Blueberry and Greens Shake**                              **Serves 2**

*This drink is a powerhouse of nutrients! The chlorella and spirulina are highly beneficial green foods. They are rich in nutrients like beta carotene and help to detoxify the liver. They are readily available at health food stores.*

1 cup nondairy milk
⅔ cup blueberries – fresh or frozen
2 tablespoons protein powder
½ teaspoon chlorella
½ teaspoon spirulina
Sprinkle of Truvia (optional)

In a blender puree the nondairy milk and blueberries. Add the rest of the ingredients and blend well.

**Simple Flax Smoothie**                                    **Serves 2**

*Flaxseed is not only a tasty addition to smoothies but it is also very nutritious. Flaxseed is high in mood balancing essential fatty acids, calcium, magnesium, and potassium.*

1 cup vanilla nondairy milk
2 tablespoons ground flaxseed
1 banana

Combine all ingredients in a blender. Blend until smooth and serve.

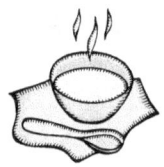

## *Healthy, Quick Breakfasts*

Most American breakfasts include wheat and dairy products, such as wheat toast, wheat cereal with milk, sweet rolls, cheese, cream cheese and other wheat- and dairy-based foods. As I explained earlier in this book, dairy products and wheat can worsen the symptoms of stress and anxiety in many women. Gluten and casein, the proteins found in wheat and milk, can trigger symptoms of mood imbalances, bloating, digestive disturbances and fatigue.

I have included in this section both whole grain, carbohydrate-based entrees as well as protein-rich breakfast dishes, depending on the type of diet that makes you feel your best. Both types of entrees, however, will benefit anxiety and stress symptoms by eliminating wheat and dairy products at breakfast.

The whole grain dishes are based on ground flaxseed, gluten-free grains and soy (if tolerated), all of which can be useful in reducing your symptoms. The protein-rich entrees have been created using eggs and healthy breakfast meats. The smoothies also contain protein powder.

**Quinoa Cereal with Raspberries**                                   **Serves 2**

1 ½ cups cooked quinoa
1 cup nondairy milk
½ cup raspberries
2 teaspoons honey or other sweetener

Combine quinoa and nondairy milk in a saucepan. Simmer for 5 minutes. Stir in honey and garnish with raspberries.

## Quinoa with Prunes Serves 2

*This is one of my all-time favorite hot cereals. The plums are delicious and add a nice texture. Quinoa is a small, protein rich grain. When cooked the grains are small and fluffy. I recommend making a pot of quinoa the night before.*

1 ½ cups cooked quinoa
1 cup nondairy milk
4-6 dried prunes, chopped
2 tablespoons flaxseed oil
2 teaspoons xylitol, honey, or maple syrup (if using unsweetened milk)
Pinch of salt (optional)

In a saucepan combine quinoa, nondairy milk, salt, and dried plums. Heat thoroughly and simmer on low heat for 5-10 minutes until plums have softened. Serve with flaxseed oil and sweetener.


## Maple Cinnamon Oatmeal Serves 2

1 cup gluten-free quick oats
1 ¾ cups water
1-2 tablespoons flaxseed oil
2 teaspoons maple syrup
Pinch of cinnamon (to taste)
Pinch of salt

Boil water in a saucepan. Add gluten-free oats and reduce to medium heat. Cook for one minute and stir. Cover, and remove oatmeal from heat. Serve in 2-3 minutes.

Stir in maple syrup, flaxseed oil, cinnamon and salt.

## Strawberries and Cream Oatmeal                    Serves 2

1 cup gluten-free quick oats
½ cup strawberries, chopped
½ nondairy milk
1 ¼ cups water
1-2 tablespoons flaxseed oil
2 teaspoons honey or stevia
Pinch of salt (optional)

Bring water and nondairy milk to a boil in a saucepan. Add gluten-free
oats and reduce to medium heat. Cook for one minute and stir. Cover, and
remove oatmeal from heat. Serve in 2-3 minutes. Stir in sweetener, flaxseed
oil, salt and top with strawberries.


## Banana Nut Muffins                    Makes 14-18

*These moist muffins are a twist on the classic recipe using cashews instead of
walnuts. Very tasty!*

1½ cups rice flour
1 teaspoon baking powder
½ teaspoon baking soda
3 ripe bananas, mashed
¼ teaspoon cinnamon
6 packets of Truvia (¼ cup)
¼ cup honey
¼ cup safflower oil
⅓ cup cashews, chopped

Preheat oven to 350 degrees. Mix all dry ingredients and wet ingredients
separately. Combine and mix well. Fill muffin cups ⅔ with the batter.

## Pumpkin Muffins

**Makes 14-18 muffins**

1½ cups rice flour
½ teaspoon baking powder
½ teaspoon baking soda
1 cup pumpkin
1 teaspoon cinnamon
¼ teaspoon nutmeg
¼ cup chopped almonds (optional)
3 tablespoons molasses
3 tablespoons safflower oil
½ cup raisins
2 eggs
½ cup nondairy milk
1 teaspoon vanilla extract
Pinch of salt

Preheat oven to 400 degrees. Line a muffin tin with paper muffin cups.

Combine all dry ingredients and mix thoroughly. In a separate bowl beat the two eggs and then combine the remainder of the wet ingredients. Add the wet ingredients to the dry and mix thoroughly.

Fill muffin cups ⅔ with the batter. Cook for 18-20 minutes or until thoroughly cooked.

**Flaxseed Pancakes**                                    **Makes 8 pancakes (serves 2-4)**

*Xylitol is an excellent sugar substitute for cooking and baking that can be found at most health food stores. Xylitol is easy to use because it has a 1:1 ratio with sugar. Yet, this product has 40% fewer calories than sugar and is beneficial for your teeth and gums. It also helps to balance your blood sugar level so doesn't trigger anxiety and mood symptoms related to blood sugar issues.*

1 cup gluten-free flour
1 cup unsweetened rice milk
1 egg
2 tablespoons xylitol
1 tablespoon ground flaxseed
1 teaspoon baking powder
½ teaspoon baking soda
¼ teaspoon salt
3 tablespoons almond oil, keeping 1 tbsp. for cooking
Maple syrup (optional)
Fruit jam (optional)

Mix the dry and wet ingredients in separate bowls. Combine all the ingredients and mix thoroughly. Cook on medium heat and use a small amount of oil to grease the pan if needed. When pancakes bubble in the center flip and cook for 1-2 minutes until cooked thoroughly. Serve with maple syrup or all-fruit jam. Delicious!

## Egg and Sausage Scramble                                    **Serves 2**

4 eggs
4 turkey breakfast sausages
2 slices of gluten-free toast
Salt and pepper (optional)
2 teaspoons olive oil
Serve with ½ cup applesauce

Warm a frying pan on medium heat and add olive oil. Beat egg gently in a small bowl and set aside. Chop the sausages into small pieces - this will help them to cook faster. Add sausages to the pan and cook for several minutes until sausages are brown. Turn heat to low and add eggs to the pan and scramble with the sausage. Add a pinch of salt and pepper. Serve with toast and applesauce.

Bake for 20-25 minutes until cooked through.


## Mushroom Onion Scramble                                    **Serves 2**

*The mushrooms and onion give this egg scramble a great texture. The water helps make the eggs fluffier.*

4 eggs
1 tablespoon water
¼ onion
2-3 mushrooms
1 tablespoon olive oil
Salt and pepper (optional)

Dice the mushrooms and onion. Next, beat the 4 eggs together with 1 tablespoon water. Preheat the frying pan on medium heat and add 1 tablespoon olive oil. Add onion and mushroom and cook for about 3 minutes until onions are translucent and add eggs. Let sit for about 30 second and then start to scramble with your spatula. Add a pinch of salt and pepper and serve.

**Spinach and Tomato Scramble**                                         **Serves 2**

*The sprinkle of Parmesan cheese adds a delightful saltiness and tang to this dish.*

4 eggs, beaten
1 tablespoon water
2 tablespoons diced onion
¼ tomato, chopped
12 spinach leaves, chopped
1 tablespoon olive oil
Salt and pepper (optional)
Parmesan cheese - or soy Parmesan (optional)

Beat the 4 eggs together with 1 tablespoon water. Preheat the frying pan on medium heat and add 1 tablespoon olive oil. Add onion and cook for about 3 minutes until onions are translucent. Next add eggs, spinach and tomato. Let sit for about 15 seconds and then start to scramble with your spatula. Sprinkle on a small amount of Parmesan cheese, add a pinch of salt and pepper and serve

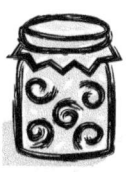 *Spreads and Sauces*

These spreads and sauces contain highly concentrated levels of ingredients that help to relax mood and muscle tension and promote hormonal balance. Serve with rice cakes, crackers, corn bread, or even spread on a banana for a delicious treat.

**Fresh Applesauce**                                               **Serves 2**

2 ½ apples
½ cup fresh apple juice
½ teaspoon cinnamon
½ teaspoon ginger

Peel apples and cut into quarters; remove cores. Combine all ingredients in a food processor. Blend until smooth.

**Sesame-Tofu Spread**                                             **Serves 4**

¼ cup soft tofu
¼ cup raw sesame butter
¼ cup honey

Combine all ingredients in a blender. Serve with rice cakes or crackers.

## Lunch and Dinner Recipes

These high-nutrient, healthful lunch and dinner dishes are designed to help relieve anxiety and balance your mood. The ingredients do not include sugar, alcohol, caffeine, additives, red meat, dairy products, or wheat, all of which can worsen your symptoms. Mix and match these dishes as you please. You might combine soups and salads or whole grains, legumes and vegetables for a complete vegetarian emphasis or enjoy a meat-based meal, depending on your needs for carbohydrates and protein.

The main course dishes are all extremely healthful for women who are trying to recover from anxiety, stress and panic attacks. They will support your health and well-being, and your family will enjoy and benefit from these dishes, too.

 *Soups*

**Split Pea Soup** Serves 4

¾ cup split peas
5 cups low-sodium chicken broth
⅔ cup carrot, chopped
¾ cup onion, diced
Tamari soy sauce – to taste (optional)

Bring the water to a boil and add the split peas, onion, carrots, and chicken broth. Reduce heat to low and simmer for 50-60 minutes, stirring occasionally. If water begins to cook off add up to an extra cup of water. Add a dash of tamari soy sauce for a saltier flavor.

## Black Bean Soup

**Serves 4**

*This recipe is easy and makes a delicious, filling soup.*

1 can black beans (14 ounce), rinsed
5 cups low-sodium vegetable broth
1 cup onion, diced
⅔ cup carrot, chopped
⅔ cup red pepper, chopped
¼ teaspoon cumin
Tamari soy sauce – to taste (optional)

Bring the water to a boil and add all ingredients. Reduce heat to low and simmer for 30 minutes, stirring occasionally. If water begins to cook off add up to an extra cup of water. Add a dash of tamari soy sauce for a saltier flavor.

## Chicken Rice Soup

**Serves 4-6**

*Few things make me feel better than a bowl of homemade chicken rice soup. I have an easy tip to add extra flavor to your soup: If you used the meat from a roasted, skin-on chicken you can add some of the skin to the soup while it is cooking. This will add depth and richness to your soup. Remove the skin when the soup has finished cooking.*

6 cups low-sodium chicken broth
⅔ cup carrot
1 cup celery, diced
1 cup cooked chicken, diced
⅔ cup onion, diced
⅔ cup brown rice, cooked
Tamari soy sauce – to taste (optional)

Bring water to a boil and add all ingredients. Reduce heat to low and simmer for 30 minutes, stirring occasionally. If water begins to cook off add up to an extra cup of water. Add a dash of tamari soy sauce for a saltier flavor.

**Butternut Squash Soup**                                          **Serves 4**

*This soup has been a long-time favorite of mine. I adore the light, creamy texture. Adding a touch of maple syrup enhances the natural sweetness of the squash.*

½ onion, diced
1 cup low-sodium chicken broth
2 cups pureed butternut squash - fresh or frozen (fresh is preferred)
½ teaspoon cinnamon
1½ cups nondairy milk
2 teaspoons maple syrup
1 tablespoon safflower oil
½-¾ teaspoon salt

In a large saucepan heat the oil on medium heat. Add the onion and cook until translucent. Add the butternut squash, chicken broth, cinnamon and salt. Mix well and simmer for 5 minutes. Add nondairy milk and maple syrup. Simmer on low heat for ten minutes. Stir frequently while cooking the soup. *Optional*: To make extra creamy, blend the soup when it has finished cooking. Wait for the soup to cool before blending.

 *Salads*

**Classic Spinach Salad** **Serves 4**

*My tip for cooking great turkey bacon is to cook it on medium-low heat. It takes a few extra minutes but is definitely worth it!*

1 bunch of spinach, approximately 6 cups
4 slices of turkey bacon, cooked crisp and crumbled
2 eggs, sliced or chopped
½ cup red pepper, chopped
¼ red onion, sliced very thin
¾ cup mushrooms, sliced thin
Balsamic-vinaigrette dressing

In a large bowl place the bacon, egg, red pepper, onion, and mushrooms on top of the spinach. Before serving, add dressing and toss the salad.

**Zingy Watercress Salad** **Serves 4**

*I enjoy the refreshing bitterness of watercress. This salad pairs well with green apple. Watercress has a strong flavor and a little goes a long way.*

1 cup watercress, coarsely chopped
4 cups butter lettuce (or other soft lettuce), coarsely chopped
2 teaspoons scallions, finely chopped
½ green apple, chopped
1 ounce goat cheese, crumbled
Vinaigrette dressing

In a large bowl toss the watercress, butter lettuce, green onion, and apple together with the vinaigrette dressing (to taste). On top of the salad crumble the goat cheese.

**Potato Salad with Vinaigrette Dressing**                    Serves 4-6

10-12 small red potatoes, cut into bite size pieces (about 2 cups)
2 tablespoons diced celery
2 tablespoons diced red onion
2 tablespoons diced red pepper
1 heaping tablespoon diced water chestnuts
1 hardboiled egg, yolk removed
Vinaigrette dressing (to taste)

Steam the potatoes for 15-20 minutes or until fork tender and let cool. Chop up all the vegetables into small pieces and set aside. Chop egg white and set aside. Toss with your favorite vinaigrette dressing.


**Scrumptious Veggie Salad**                    Serves 4-6

*This is one of my favorite salads! It pairs wonderfully with soups and sandwiches.*

1 head red lettuce, chopped into bite size pieces
1 large tomato, chopped
2 green onions, sliced
6 mushrooms, sliced
¾ cup kidney beans – canned works well
1 avocado, sliced
¼ cup sunflower seeds
Vinaigrette dressing (to taste)

Combine all ingredients except for avocado in a large salad bowl. Mix in Vinaigrette dressing and top with avocado slices before serving.

## Radicchio and Orange Salad Serves 4-6

*This is a sophisticated and delicious salad. I love salads with "extras" such as fruit or a little bit of goat cheese.*

6 cups salad greens
½ radicchio, sliced thin
⅓ red onion, sliced very thin
3 ounces goat cheese
1 medium sized orange, peeled and cut into bite size segments
Orange vinaigrette

In a large bowl combine salad greens, radicchio, onion, and oranges. Pour vinaigrette, to taste, over salad and toss. Add goat cheese before serving.

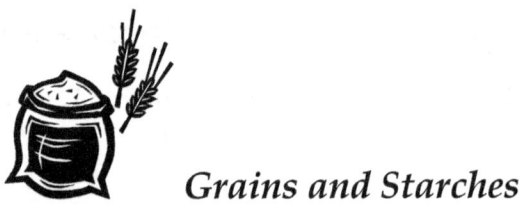

*Grains and Starches*

**Wild Rice**                                                     Serves 2

⅔ cup wild rice
2 ½ cups water
½ teaspoon salt

Wash rice with cold water. Combine all ingredients in a cooking pot and bring to a rapid boil. Turn flame to low, cover, and cook without stirring (about 45 minutes) until rice is tender but not mushy. Uncover and fluff with a fork. Cook an additional 5 minutes, and then serve.

**Kasha**                                                        Serves 4

1 cup kasha (buckwheat groats)
3 ¼ cups water
Pinch of salt

Bring ingredients to a boil, lower heat, and simmer for 25 minutes or until soft. The grains should be fluffy, like rice.

*For breakfast, blend in blender with water until creamy. Add almond milk, sesame milk, or sunflower milk, and cinnamon, apple butter, raisins, or berries.*

**Delicious Baked Sweet Potato**                                 Serves 4

4 sweet potatoes
1 teaspoon olive oil
1 tablespoon flax oil for each potato

Preheat oven to 400° F. Wash the potatoes, then rub with olive oil. Bake for 45 to 60 minutes, or until soft when pierced with a fork. Garnish with flax oil. Honey, maple syrup, or chopped raw pecans may also be used.

**Baked Potato** **Serves 4**

4 russet or Idaho potatoes
2 teaspoons olive oil
1 tablespoon flax oil for each potato

Preheat oven to 400° F. Wash the potatoes, rub them with olive oil, and bake for 45 to 60 minutes, or until soft when pierced with a fork. Garnish with flax oil.

*Other garnishes can include chopped green onions, soy cheese, and salsa.*

 *Vegetables*

## Kale with Lemon                                                        Serves 4

*Kale is one of my favorite vegetables and it also has terrific health benefits for women since it is a good source of calcium and other essential nutrients like lutein that supports healthy hormonal balance and the health of your heart and eyes.*

1 bunch of kale
1 lemon, cut into quarters
Soy sauce

Rinse kale well and remove stems. Steam for 5-6 minutes or until leaves wilt and are tender. Dress lightly with soy sauce and lemon juice.

## Simple Steamed Cabbage                                                 Serves 4

1 small head cabbage, quartered
1 teaspoon chopped parsley
1 teaspoon olive oil
Pinch of salt (optional)

Steam cabbage until tender. Sprinkle with olive oil and parsley.

## Jessica's Favorite Broccoli                                            Serves 4

1 pound broccoli
1 tablespoons flaxseed oil
Pinch of salt (optional)
Squeeze of lemon

Cut the broccoli into small florets; steam until tender. Squeeze lemon juice over broccoli and add the flax oil. Mix and serve.

## Cauliflower with Flaxseed Oil                    Serves 4

1 medium head cauliflower
2 tablespoons flaxseed oil
Pinch of salt (optional)

Break the cauliflower into small florets. Steam until tender. Toss with flax oil and salt.


## Roasted Rosemary Potatoes                    Serves 4-6

*I love roasted potatoes! This is a wonderful potato recipe that I like to make when I serve roasted chicken.*

4 cups red potatoes – about 4 or 5 large red potatoes
1 tablespoon dried rosemary, crushed
3 tablespoons of olive oil
2 garlic cloves, minced
Pinch of pepper (optional)
Pinch of salt

Preheat oven to 400 degrees. Cut potatoes into bite size pieces and put into plastic bag. Add olive oil, rosemary, garlic, and black pepper to bag. Close bag and shake to coat all of the potato pieces.

Line a baking tray with foil and put potatoes on to tray. Arrange evenly in one layer. Sprinkle salt onto potatoes and bake for 30-35 minutes until brown and cooked through. During cooking stir the potatoes once if desired.

**Honey Carrots** Serves 4

*This is one of my favorite side dishes. The touch of warm honey brings out the natural sweetness of the carrots.*

3 cups carrots, sliced thin
1 teaspoon honey
1 teaspoon almond oil
Pinch of salt (optional)

Cut carrots into thin slices and steam for 6-8 minutes, or until tender. Using the same saucepan pour out the cooking water and on low heat add the honey and oil and mix well. Add carrots and mix all ingredients together. Add a pinch of salt before serving.

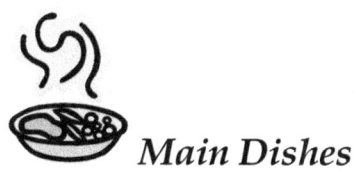 *Main Dishes*

**Mega Greens Rice Bowl** **Serves 4**

*This dish is a satisfying way to get a large serving of healthy greens. A delicious sauce is Organicville's Island Teriyaki (organicvillefoods.com). Their sauce is made with agave nectar instead of cane sugar.*

4 cups kale, cut into bite size pieces (about ½ bunch)
3 cups baby bok choy, chopped
1 cup of white mushrooms, sliced
1 carrot, finely chopped
8 ounces of tofu, cubed
3 cups cooked brown rice - ¾ cup rice per person
Teriyaki sauce – soy sauce - gomasio

Steam the carrots for 4 minutes and then add the kale, bok choy, mushrooms, and tofu. Steam for 5 minutes. Serve in a deep bowl over rice with your choice of sauce.

Good sauces for this dish include teriyaki sauce and soy sauce. A little bit of lemon juice and gomasio also works well.

**Baked Tofu Rice Bowl**                                    **Serves 4**

*Baked tofu has a rich, nutty flavor that I love. This recipe is fun but also very tasty and rich in healthy greens. I always make sure that the vegetables are cut into bite size pieces.*

3 cups broccoli, chopped
3 cups baby bok choy, chopped
1 carrot, finely chopped
½ cup mushrooms, sliced
½ cup red pepper
Baked tofu
3 cups cooked brown rice - ¾ cup rice per person

Steam the carrots for 4 minutes and then add the broccoli, baby bok choy, mushrooms, and red pepper. Steam for 5 minutes. Serve in a deep bowl over rice with your choice of sauce. Layer a few pieces of baked tofu on top.

**Summertime Veggie Pasta**                                 **Serves 4**

*This light pasta is one of my favorite dishes to eat during the summer. The pasta and sauce are light but filling. It's a dish that I love to share to share with friends.*

1 box quinoa elbow pasta (8 ounce box)
½ onion, diced
2 cans Italian seasoned diced tomatoes
1 can garbanzo beans
1 carrot, shredded
1½ cups cooked Brussels sprouts or broccoli
½ teaspoon dried basil
2 teaspoons olive oil
Pinch of pepper
Pinch of salt (optional)

Cook pasta according to package directions. In a saucepan on medium heat add olive oil and onions. Sautee until onions are translucent. Add remainder of ingredients and bring to a simmer. Cook on low heat for 10 minutes. Combine the cooked noodles with the sauce.

**Eggplant Parmesan** **Serves 4-6**

*I love eggplant Parmesan. It is a rich and extremely delicious entree. This version, while wonderful, takes a little more time and has a few more steps than most of my entrees. Even though I use substitutions for the cheese, the dish is still very rich and I recommend saving it for a special occasion or party. You will wow your guests with how tasty it is! My favorite non-dairy cheese alternative is sold by Follow Your Heart. Their products can be found in health food stores or at followyourheart.com*

1 eggplant, cut into ⅓ - ½ inch slices (peeling is optional)
2 eggs, beaten
1 ¼ cups gluten-free breadcrumbs
3 cups of pasta sauce, tomato and basil flavor
8 ounces of mozzarella cheese, shredded
⅓ cup Parmesan or soy Parmesan cheese, grated
¼ cup olive oil - divided

Arrange the eggplant slices in a colander or on a rack placed over the sink. Sprinkle all of the slices generously with salt and let stand 30 minutes; the eggplant slices will release water. Rinse and pat dry. Next, dip each slice in the beaten egg and coat with breadcrumbs.

Heat a portion of the olive oil in a skillet over medium heat. Cook the eggplant until golden on each side, about 2-3 minutes. If necessary, reduce the heat to medium-low. Repeat until all of the eggplant is cooked.

Preheat the oven 350°. Arrange half the eggplant slices on the bottom of a lightly oiled baking dish (a 9x9 or 9x12 pan works well). Spread half of the pasta sauce on top. Sprinkle with half of the mozzarella and half of the Parmesan cheese. Repeat with the next layer.

Bake 25-30 minutes or until mixture is bubbly.

**Parmesan Chicken Pasta**                                    **Serves 4**

*This dish is a crowd pleaser that I often serve when I have friends over. The sprinkle of Parmesan cheese adds a delightful tanginess that rounds out the dish perfectly.*

6 cups gluten-free pasta, cooked
1 ½ cups roasted chicken, cubed
⅔ cup diced carrots
⅔ cup diced red onion
½ onion, diced
1 small tomato, finely chopped
3 cups broccoli, chopped into bite size pieces
⅔ cup chicken broth (recommended) or water
1 teaspoon dried basil
1 tablespoon olive oil
Soy Parmesan cheese or regular, grated
Generous pinch of pepper
Pinch of salt (optional)

In a frying pan on medium heat add the olive oil. Add the onion and sauté until onion begins to turn translucent. Add all vegetables except tomatoes and cook for 1-2 minutes. Add chicken broth, chicken, tomatoes, basil, and pepper. Turn heat to low, cover and simmer for 5-7 minutes or until broth has cooked down. Add more broth if needed.

Add the sauce to the pasta. Serve with Parmesan cheese.


**Simple Broiled Tuna**                                       **Serves 4**

4 fillets of tuna, 4 ounces each
2 teaspoons olive oil
Squeeze of lemon juice
Pinch of salt

Baste the tuna fillets with oil; then sprinkle with lemon juice. Place tuna in a broiler pan and broil until the level of doneness that you prefer (rare or well-done).

**Simple Steamed Salmon**                                    **Serves 4**

4 fillets of salmon, 4 ounces each
1 cup water
Squeeze of lemon

Combine water and lemon juice in a steamer. Place salmon fillets in streamer basket. Cook to the level of doneness that you prefer.


**Turkey Bolognese**                                     **Serves 2-4**

*This dish cooks up quickly and is very satisfying. This is a versatile recipe. You can add all kinds of vegetables and it will taste great.*

½ lb. ground turkey
2 cans of diced tomatoes
1 can tomato paste
½ onion, diced
1 carrot, diced
1 zucchini, diced
1 teaspoon basil
1 teaspoon oregano
1 tablespoon olive oil
¼ teaspoon salt (optional)
½ teaspoon pepper (optional)
Water (optional)

Heat pan on medium and add olive oil. Add onion and sauté until translucent. Add turkey and all herbs and spices. Cook until turkey has browned and cooked thoroughly. Add tomatoes, tomato paste, carrots, and zucchini. Cook on low heat for 12-15 minutes. If sauce is too thick add a small amount of water until desired consistency is reached. Serve over brown rice spaghetti.

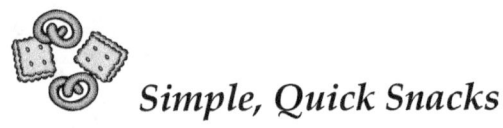 *Simple, Quick Snacks*

**Trail Mix**                                    Makes ¾ cup

¼ cup raw unsalted pumpkin seeds
¼ cup raw unsalted sunflower seeds
¼ cup raisins

Combine and store in a container in the refrigerator. This trail mix is very high in essential fatty acids, calcium, magnesium, and iron that help to balance your brain chemistry, moods and hormones. I use it for a snack food to replace stressful and unhealthy sugar-based sweets and chocolate. It is a great mix to take on trips, and I eat it often for breakfast.

**Rice Cakes with Nut Butter and Jam**                    Serves 2

4 unsalted rice cakes
2 tablespoons raw almond butter
2 tablespoons fruit preserves (no sugar added)

Spread rice cakes with almond butter and fruit preserves for a quick snack.

*Herbal tea makes a good accompaniment.*

**Rice Cakes with Tuna Fish**                             Serves 2

4 unsalted rice cakes
4 ounces tuna fish
2 teaspoons low-calorie mayonnaise

Spread rice cakes with tuna fish and mayonnaise.

*This is an excellent high-protein, high-carbohydrate snack.*

## Apple with Almond Butter

**Serves 2**

1 apple, sliced
1 tablespoon raw almond butter

Spread almond butter on thin apple slices.


## Banana with Sesame Butter

**Serves 2**

1 banana, halved
1 tablespoon raw sesame butter

Spread sesame butter on each half of a ripe banana.

# Healthy Food Shopping List

## Vegetables

| | | |
|---|---|---|
| Beets | Eggplant | Radicchio |
| Bok choy | Garlic | Radishes |
| Broccoli | Green beans | Rutabagas |
| Brussels sprouts | Horseradish | Sauerkraut |
| Cabbage | Kale | Spinach |
| Carrots | Lettuce | Squash |
| Cauliflower | Mustard greens | Sweet potatoes |
| Celery | Okra | Tomatoes |
| Chard | Onions | Turnips |
| Cilantro | Parsley | Turnip greens |
| Collard | Parsnips | Watercress |
| Cucumbers | Peas (all varieties) | Yams |
| Dandelion greens | Potatoes | |

| **Legumes** | **Whole Grains** | **Seeds and Nuts** |
|---|---|---|
| Adzuki | Amaranth | Almonds |
| Black | Barley | Cashews |
| Black-eyed peas | Brown rice | Filberts |
| Cannellini | Buckwheat | Flaxseeds |
| Fava | Corn | Macadamia |
| Garbanzo | Millet | Pecan |
| Kidney | Oatmeal | Pumpkin seeds |
| Lentils | Quinoa | Sesame seeds |
| Navy | Rye | Sunflower seeds |
| Red | | Walnuts |
| Soy: tofu, tempeh | | |
| Turtle beans | | |

## Healthy Food Shopping List (continued)

### Fruits
Acai berries
Apples
Avocado
Bananas
Berries (like blueberries, raspberries, or strawberries)
Coconuts
Goji berries
Kiwi
Noni
Olives
Pomegranates
Pears
Seasonal fruits (one per day)

### Sweeteners
brown rice syrup
honey
maple syrup
molasses
stevia
xylitol

### Beverages
Coconut water
Grain based coffee substitute
Herbal tea
Green tea
Water

### Meats
Fish
Free-range poultry
Game meat
Organic lean red meat
Seafood (in moderation)

### Oils
Flax
Macadamia
Olive
Safflower
Sesame
Walnut

### Foods from Other Cultures
Gomasio
Jicama
Miso
Seaweed (like kelp, dulse, nori, wakane)
Tamari soy sauce
Umeboshi plums

### Dairy Substitutes
Hemp milk
Nut milk
Rice milk
Soy milk
Soy, coconut, almond, rice or hemp cheeses, cream cheese, yogurt, and frozen desserts
*Avoid all soy products containing hydrogenated oil.

### Herbs & Spices
Basil
Black pepper
Cayenne pepper
Chamomile
Chili pepper, dried
Cilantro
Cinnamon, ground
Cloves
Coriander
Cumin
Dill
Ginger
Licorice
Mustard seeds
Oregano
Peppermint
Poppy
Rosemary
Sage
Tarragon
Thyme
Turmeric

# 7

# Vitamins, Minerals, Herbs & Essential Fatty Acids

During my years of working with patients, I have found that the use of therapeutic nutritional supplements can play a very important role in the treatment and prevention of anxiety and panic episodes. In this chapter, I share with you essential information about the most beneficial nutrients that can support your anxiety and stress recovery program.

The right mix of nutrients can help to support healthy brain and nervous system chemistry so that feelings of anxiety and fear do not get triggered in such an intense way when dealing with life's stresses. Therapeutic nutrients can help to create a greater sense of peace and calm and a more balanced mood as you go through your busy day. They can promote deep, peaceful restful sleep if you are struggling with sleeplessness and insomnia when you are feeling more anxious.

Nutritional supplements can also improve your ability to manage stress by supporting your general health and well-being. They can improve the functioning of your immune system, endocrine glands, and digestive tract. They can also stimulate healthy circulation of blood and oxygen to the entire body, including your brain, which further benefits your mood and is necessary for high energy and vitality. Numerous research studies that have been done at university centers and hospitals support the importance of nutrition in promoting all of these benefits for your mood and general health.

Even with an excellent diet, it is difficult to take in the therapeutic levels of nutrients needed for optimal healing from anxiety, stress and panic attacks. The use of nutritional supplements can help bridge this gap so you feel better as rapidly and completely as possible. I do want to, however, emphasize the importance of a good diet along with the use of supplements. Supplements should never be used as an excuse to continue poor dietary habits. I have found that my patients heal most effectively when they combine a nutrient-rich diet with the right mix of supplements.

In this chapter, I share with you the best nutritional supplements to achieve these goals. The chapter is divided into five sections. The first two discuss the most effective amino acids, vitamins and minerals for relieving anxiety and stress symptoms; the third section discusses the best herbs to help relieve anxiety. The fourth section explains the benefits of essential fatty acids.

Finally, I conclude the chapter with a chart that summarizes all of the nutritional supplements that I discuss in the first four sections as well as recommendations on how to best use nutritional supplements. I also provide you with a sample nutritional supplement formula and a series of charts that list major food sources for each essential nutrient.

As you read through the chapter, I suggest that you consider using the supplements that are most targeted towards your specific set of symptoms. You may also have specific preferences about the types of supplements that you would like to use. For example, some women are more interested in correcting imbalances in brain chemistry through the use of amino acids while others are drawn more towards using herbs.

I suggest that you begin by using the types of nutritional supplements that you feel most drawn towards that I discuss in this chapter. Vitamins and minerals can often be taken in combination by using a high potency multinutrient product. Nutritional supplements are readily available in health food stores or can be ordered through the Internet.

Remember that all women differ somewhat in their nutritional needs. If you do take the recommended vitamin or herbal supplements, I usually advise that you start with one-fourth to one-half the dose recommended in this book and work your way up slowly to the higher dosage, if needed. You may find that you do best with slightly more or less of certain ingredients.

Let's begin now by looking at the different types of nutritional supplements that can provide the greatest relief of anxiety and stress symptoms!

## Amino Acids for Relief of Anxiety

There are two crucial neurotransmitter pathways that help to support balance within your brain as well as your overall health and well-being. The first leads to the production of inhibitory neurotransmitters such as serotonin and GABA, while the second leads to the production of excitatory neurotransmitters like dopamine, norepinephrine, and epinephrine.

Generally speaking, the inhibitor neurotransmitters quiet down the processes of your body, while the excitatory neurotransmitters stimulate them, speeding them up. Thus, the brain chemicals produced through these two pathways oppose and complement one another. When these chemicals are out of balance, you may be more prone towards anxiety and panic episodes or depression and sadness.

Women who suffer from anxiety often benefit most from nutritional supplements that support the inhibitory neurotransmitters since they have a quieting and calming effect on the brain and emotions and help to eliminate anxiety symptoms.

All neurotransmitters are derived from nutrients that you take in through your diet. They are either produced from amino acids found in the protein that you eat or can be taken as supplements. To best relieve symptoms of anxiety, stress and panic episodes, you may want to supplement with the key amino acids that I discuss in this section as well as vitamins, and minerals that help to promote their beneficial effects in your brain and nervous system.

I recommend that you read through the descriptions of these supplements and learn about their specific benefits for combatting stress. You may find that using a particular one or even combining several will best suit your needs. These nutrients can be bought individually in health food stores or through the Internet. There are also a number of products that combine these amino acids and hormones like melatonin. These combined products can produce an even stronger therapeutic effect if your anxiety symptoms tend to be more intense.

*5-HTP.* Within your brain, serotonin often inhibits the firing of neurons, which dampens many of your behaviors. In fact, serotonin has one of the most widespread effects on the brain and physiology. It plays a key role in regulating temperature, blood pressure, blood clotting, immunity, pain, digestion, sleep, and biorhythms. Serotonin also produces a relaxing effect on your mood so it can be very helpful for women who suffer from anxiety and stress.

Serotonin is produced within the body from an amino acid precursor, tryptophan, which can be taken in through the diet or as a supplement. The essential amino acid tryptophan is initially converted into an intermediary substance called 5-hydroxytryptophan (5-HTP), which is then converted into serotonin the major inhibitory neurotransmitter.

While tryptophan is available as a supplement and is abundant in turkey, pumpkin seeds, and almonds, I've found that 5-HTP is a more effective and reliable option for boosting your neurotransmitter production. 5-HTP is very helpful for women suffering from fatigue and tiredness due to sleeplessness and insomnia. Numerous double-blind studies have shown that 5-HTP is as effective as many of the more common antidepressant drugs and is associated with fewer and much milder side effects. In addition to increasing serotonin levels, 5-HTP triggers an increase in endorphins and other neurotransmitters that are often low in cases of depression when it coexists with anxiety.

To maintain proper serotonin levels, it is helpful to take 50–100 mg of 5-HTP once or twice a day, with one of the dosages taken at bedtime. Be sure to start at 50 mg and increase as necessary. If needed during the day, use carefully, as too much serotonin can interfere with your ability to drive or concentrate.

*GABA (gamma amino butric acid).* Research suggests that women with generalized anxiety disorder may have an imbalance of gamma amino butyric acid (GABA) in their brain. GABA is a neurotransmitter, a substance that transmits messages from one part of the brain to another. When people are given GABA or placed on drugs that increase the activity of GABA, their anxiety is diminished. While the exact mechanism triggering the generalized anxiety is not known, it is possible that a GABA deficiency or extreme sensitivity on the part of the body to the available GABA levels may play a role in its etiology. I recommend 250 to 500 mg of GABA two to three times per day for anxiety. For insomnia, 500 mg of GABA can be taken before bedtime. GABA should be taken on an empty stomach.

*Taurine*. This substance helps to promote feelings of peace and calm and prevent overactivity of the excitatory neurotransmitters. It helps to support restful sleep and is useful in the control of anxiety and bipolar disorder. It also helps to control seizure disorders. Taurine helps to move important minerals like potassium, calcium and magnesium in and out of the heart, thereby enhancing heart health. As a sulfur containing amino acid, it also helps in the process of detoxification. It conjugates or binds with bile acids to maintain the solubility of fats and cholesterol in bile, thereby helping to prevent the formation of gallstones. A standard dosage of Taurine is 1000 – 3000 mg a day.

*L-Theanine or theanine*. It is an amino acid that is found mainly in green tea plants. Research studies suggest that theanine is beneficial in the treatment of anxiety and stress symptoms. It has a peaceful and calming effect on the mood and the physical functions of the body, including reduction of heart rate. Heart rate is often increased during anxiety and panic episodes. Theanine may even lessen the intensity of the "fight or flight" response commonly seen with high levels of stress. Another benefit of theanine is that it helps to promote alpha waves within the brain. Alpha brain waves cycle between 8 to 12 Hz which is seen with a relaxed brain state. In contrast, beta brain waves cycle more rapidly and are seen in states of mental arousal and higher level of activity and busyness. The standard theanine dosage is usually between 50 to 250 mg per day.

*Melatonin*. This is a hormone produced from serotonin and secreted by the pineal gland. Its secretion takes place at night and is inhibited by light. As such, it sets and regulates the timing of your body's natural circadian rhythms, such as waking and sleeping. Unfortunately, as you get older, you produce less and less melatonin. This is due, in part, to menopause. Women who have poor sleep patterns, such as night shift workers, are also more likely to have decreased melatonin production. Finally, women who suffer from anxiety, panic attacks and phobias may also have sleep disturbances and insomnia due to melatonin imbalances. I have seen women as young as their twenties and thirties benefit from melatonin supplementation, if they were prone to anxiety and panic episodes.

To ensure that you have adequate levels of melatonin, I suggest supplementing with 0.3 to 1 mg at bedtime. Paradoxically, less is often better than a higher dosage. In fact, the most effective dosage appears to be .3 mg. To help ensure that you sleep through the night, you may want to take melatonin as a time released capsule. However, some women may find that they do better with a higher dosage. In this case, I suggest taking 1.5 – 3 mg.

For melatonin to be effective, your bedroom should be dark, as light suppresses its release. Drugs such as aspirin, ibuprofen, beta-blockers, calcium channel blocks, sleeping pills and tranquilizer may deplete melatonin levels.

## Vitamins and Minerals for Relief of Anxiety

Many vitamins and minerals are useful in the treatment and prevention of anxiety, stress and panic attacks. They are also necessary for the best results when using amino acids to support neurotransmitter production within the brain. This section contains complete information on those supplements that provide the most symptom relief.

While I discuss each vitamin and mineral supplement separately, you will probably be able to take most of them together in a high quality, multinutrient product. Good products are available in health food stores and through the Internet. I provide a sample product formula for you at the end of this chapter.

*Vitamin B-Complex.* This complex consists of 11 separate B vitamins that are often found together in food. In many cases they participate in the same chemical reactions in the body; therefore, they need to be taken together for the best results. The B vitamins play an important role in healthy nervous system function. Many of them are needed to ensure a healthy brain chemistry and optimal balance between your inhibitory neurotransmitters like serotonin and your excitatory neurotransmitters like dopamine. When one or more of these vitamins are deficient, symptoms of nervous system impairment as well as anxiety, stress, and fatigue can result. Conversely, adequate intake of these nutrients can help to calm the mood and provide important components for a stable and consistent source of brain energy.

B-complex vitamins also help regulate the mood and emotional well-being, by facilitating carbohydrate metabolism and the cellular conversion of glucose to usable energy (ATP). Certain B vitamins help promote cell respiration, so the cells can use oxygen efficiently. In addition, B vitamins are needed for healthy liver function. When they are deficient, the liver is unable to efficiently perform its role as the body's chief detoxifying organ. This role includes the inactivation of estrogen. When excessive levels of estrogen accumulate in the body, it acts as a brain stimulant, worsening symptoms of anxiety and nervous tension. B vitamins are also necessary to enable the liver to detoxify alcohol. Excessive alcohol consumption can deplete vitamin B12 and folic acid as well as other vitamins in the B family and affect both your mood and level of energy.

Deficiencies of individual B vitamins can increase anxiety and stress symptoms. Pantothenic acid (vitamin B5) is needed for healthy adrenal function. High emotional stress triggers the fight-or-flight alarm response in the body, which includes excessive output of adrenal hormones, thereby worsening anxiety.

Pyridoxine (vitamin B6) also affects moods through its important role in the conversion of linoleic acid to gamma-linolenic acid (GLA) in the production of the beneficial series-1 prostaglandins. Prostaglandins have a relaxant effect on both mood and smooth muscle tissue. Lack of these relaxant hormones has been linked to PMS-related anxiety, mood swings and irritability as well as menstrual cramps, and stress-related problems like irritable bowel syndrome and migraine headaches.

Using the birth control pill, which is a common treatment for PMS, menstrual cramps and menstrual irregularity, can decreases vitamin B6 levels. Menopausal women on estrogen replacement therapy are also at risk of B6 deficiency. Anxiety symptoms can occur as a side effect of hormone use in both groups of women, in part because of B6 deficiency. B6 supplementation may help reduce these symptoms. B6 can be safely used in doses up to 150 mg. Doses above this level can be neurotoxic and should be avoided.

Lack of B6 may also increase anxiety symptoms directly through its effect on the nervous system. B6 is needed for the conversion of the amino acid tryptophan to serotonin, an important neurotransmitter. Serotonin regulates sleep, and when it is deficient, insomnia occurs. Sleeplessness is a condition often seen in women suffering from anxiety. Serotonin levels also strongly affect mood and social behavior. Both B6 and food sources of tryptophan such as almonds, pumpkin seeds, sesame seeds, and certain other protein-containing foods are necessary for adequate serotonin production.

For those women who fall asleep easily but can't return to sleep after awakening in the middle of the night, niacin (vitamin B3) may be helpful. Research studies have shown that niacinamide, a form of niacin, has effects similar to those of the minor tranquilizers. You can take between 50 to 500 mg but I recommend taking it at the lower dosage range. Above 500 mg, niacinamide can cause abnormalities in the liver enzymes.

Vitamin B12 deficiency has been linked to both anxiety and depression. Many symptoms of vitamin B12 deficiency are typical of those seen with anxiety including irritability, rapid heartbeat, chest pain, dizziness, fatigue, feeling hyperactive or frenetic, difficulty concentrating, tingling sensation in the hands and feet and cold hands and feet.

B12 is found mainly in animal foods such as lean red meats, poultry, fish and dairy products like yogurt and cheese. Women following a vegan diet (a vegetarian diet utilizing no dairy products or eggs) should take particular care to add supplemental vitamin B12 to their diets. Vitamin B12 deficiency can also occur if you lack an enzyme called intrinsic factor that helps to absorb B12 during the process of digestion in the small intestines.

I recommend B12 dosages between 250 to 1000 mcg. You may want to take dosages as high as 1000 to 2000 mcg initially for the treatment of anxiety symptoms for several weeks and then reduce your dosage to a maintenance level of 500 to 1000 mcg. B12 supplements are available as oral tablets and sprays.

In summary, the entire range of B vitamins are needed to provide nutritional support for the relief of anxiety and stress symptoms. Because B vitamins are water soluble, the body cannot readily store them. Thus, B vitamins must be taken in daily in the diet. Women who are anxious and experiencing significant stress should eat foods high in B vitamins and use vitamin supplements. Good sources of most B vitamins include whole grain germ and bran, beans, peas, nuts, brewer's yeast (which many women cannot digest readily) and liver. B12 is found mainly in animal foods. Women following a vegan diet (a vegetarian diet utilizing no dairy products or eggs) should take particular care to add supplemental vitamin B12 to their diets.

*Vitamin C.* This is an extremely important anti-stress nutrient that can help decrease the fatigue symptoms that often accompany excessive levels of anxiety and stress. It is also needed for the production of neuro-transmitters within the brain and for adrenal gland hormones. When the fight-or-flight pattern is activated in response to stress, these hormones become depleted. Larger amounts of vitamin C in the diet are needed when stress levels are high. In one research study done on 411 dentists and their spouses, scientists found a clear relationship between lack of vitamin C and the presence of fatigue.

By supporting the immune function, vitamin C helps prevent fatigue caused by infections. It stimulates the production of interferon, a chemical that prevents the spread of viruses in the body. Necessary for healthy white blood cells and their antibody production, vitamin C also helps the body fight bacterial and fungal infections. Women with low vitamin C intake tend to have elevated levels of histamine, a chemical that triggers allergy symptoms. Allergy attacks can be the cause of emotional symptoms like anxiety.

Vitamin C has also been tested, along with bioflavonoids, as a treatment for anemia caused by heavy menstrual bleeding—a common cause of fatigue and depression in teenagers and pre-menopausal women in their forties. Vitamin C reduces bleeding by helping to strengthen capillaries and prevent capillary fragility.

One clinical study of vitamin C showed a reduction in bleeding in 87 percent of women taking supplemental amounts of this essential nutrient. By strengthening the capillaries, vitamin C improves the metabolism of all the systems in the body. Healthy blood vessels permit better flow of nutrients into the cells, as well as facilitating the flow of waste products out of the cells. This is necessary for optimal health and well-being.

The best sources of vitamin C in nature are fruits and vegetables. It is a water-soluble vitamin, so it is not stored in the body. Thus, women with anxiety and excessive stress should replenish their vitamin C supply daily through a healthy diet and the use of supplements. I recommend 1000 to 3000 mg per day of mineral buffered vitamin C, taken in divided doses.

*Bioflavonoids.* In nature, bioflavonoids often occur with vitamin C in fruits and vegetables. They are abundant in citrus fruits, especially in the pulp and the white rind. They are also found in buckwheat. Along with vitamin C, bioflavonoids strengthen the cells of small blood vessels and prevent anemia due to heavy menstrual bleeding, a common cause of fatigue and depression.

Certain bioflavonoids belong to a classification of estrogen-containing plants called "phytoestrogens." Other plants in this group include fennel, anise, and licorice. Though these plants are estrogenic, they are much weaker than the hormones prescribed by doctors. These plant sources of estrogen can compete with the estrogen precursors produced by your body for space on the binding sites of enzymes needed for estrogen production. Thus, on one hand, bioflavonoids can lower excessive estrogen levels that trigger PMS and other health problems such as fibroids and endometriosis.

On the other hand, the weakly estrogenic effect of the bioflavonoids can actually help relieve symptoms such as hot flashes, night sweats, anxiety, mood swings, and insomnia in menopausal women grossly deficient in estrogen. One study researching the beneficial effects of bioflavonoids on menopausal women was done in Chicago at Loyola University Medical School. The study showed that bioflavonoids were very effective in decreasing hot flashes. In summary, the bioflavonoids actually help to normalize estrogen levels in a variety of gynecological conditions. This can help decrease symptoms of anxiety and stress that are linked to hormonal imbalances. I recommend 800 to 2500 mg per day of bioflavonoids taken as a supplement.

*Soy Isoflavones.* Like bioflavonoids, these are weakly estrogen-like substances. They are found abundantly in soybeans and can help to balance hormones and regulate mood swings and anxiety in peri-menopausal and menopausal women. They are available as capsules or in powder form. Therapeutic dosages are 50 to 100 mg per day.

*Vitamin E.* Like bioflavonoids, vitamin E relieves symptoms of anxiety and mood swings triggered by an estrogen-progesterone imbalance. This can occur in women suffering from either PMS or menopause. In studies of vitamin E as an alternative treatment for menopause, it has relieved hot flashes, night sweats, mood swings, and even vaginal dryness. Women who find that conventional estrogen therapy actually worsens their anxiety symptoms (because the available drug doses do not match their body's needs) are also potentially good candidates for vitamin E therapy.

In women suffering from PMS, vitamin E helped alleviate anxiety, mood swings, and food craving symptoms. In several controlled studies, it has also been found to help reduce fibrocystic breast lumps and breast tenderness.

Vitamin E is a very important nutrient for women's health. The best natural sources of vitamin E are wheat germ oil, walnut oil, soy bean oil, and other grain and seed oils. I generally recommend that women with menopause and PMS-related anxiety use between 400 to 1600 I.U. per day. Women with hypertension, diabetes, or bleeding problems should start on a much lower dose of vitamin E (100 I.U. per day). If you have any of these conditions, ask your physician about the advisability of using these supplements. Any increase in dosage should be made slowly and monitored carefully in these women. Otherwise, vitamin E tends to be extremely safe and is commonly used by millions of people.

*Magnesium.* This essential mineral is involved in over 300 enzymatic reactions in our bodies and is essential for healthy brain and nervous system functioning. It helps to calm and relax the mind through its role in the synthesis of neurotransmitters like serotonin. It also interferes with the release of excitatory chemicals like norepinephrine and epinephrine from the adrenal medulla, which triggers the fight-or-flight response while low levels of magnesium in relationship to calcium increases the release of catecholamines, thus, intensifying the stress response.

Given the important role that magnesium plays in these brain and nervous system reactions, it is not surprising that magnesium deficiency is linked to anxiety, panic attacks, insomnia, hyperactivity, sensitivity to loud noises, restlessness, painful leg and foot cramps at night and sugar craving.

The body also requires adequate levels of magnesium in order to maintain energy and vitality. Women suffering from excessive levels of anxiety often experience increased levels of stress and wear and tear on the body and depleted energy levels. The body needs magnesium in order to produce ATP, the end product of the conversion of food to usable energy by the body's cells. ATP is the universal energy currency that the body uses to run hundreds of thousands of chemical reactions. The digestive system can efficiently extract this energy from food only in the presence of magnesium, oxygen, and other nutrients. When magnesium is deficient, ATP production falls and the body forms lactic acid, instead. Researchers have linked excessive accumulation of lactic acid with anxiety and irritability symptoms.

Magnesium is also needed to facilitate both the conversion of the essential fatty acid linoleic acid to gamma-linolenic acid and the conversion of gamma-linolenic acid to the beneficial relaxant prostaglandin hormones. Stimulating production of these hormones helps to reduce the anxiety and mood swing symptoms of PMS, eating disorders, and agoraphobia (fear of public places).

Research has found magnesium deficiencies in the red blood cells of women suffering from PMS. In one study of 192 women, magnesium nitrate was given one week premenstrually and during the first two days of menstruation. Nervous tension was relieved in 89 percent of the women studied. These women also noted relief of headaches, breast tenderness, and weight gain. Interestingly enough, deficiency of magnesium has also been found to cause signs of stress in the adrenal gland. This is noteworthy since the adrenal gland helps to mediate physiological stress in the body.

Medical research studies on the treatment of fatigue use a special form of magnesium called magnesium aspartate. It is formed by combining magnesium with aspartic acid. Aspartic acid also plays an important role in the production of energy in the body and helps transport magnesium and potassium into the cells. Magnesium aspartate, along with potassium aspartate, has been tested in a number of clinical studies and has been shown to reduce fatigue after five to six weeks of constant use. Many volunteers began to feel better even within ten days. This beneficial effect was seen in 90 percent of the people tested, a very high success rate. This could be beneficial if your anxiety and stress symptoms are causing you to feel more tired.

Magnesium is an important nutrient for women with stress-related intestinal problems, particularly irritable bowel syndrome, diarrhea and vomiting. A magnesium deficiency can develop if these symptoms are chronic. When a deficiency occurs, it can worsen anxiety, fatigue, weakness, confusion, and muscle tremor in susceptible women. Women with these symptoms must replace the magnesium through appropriate supplementation.

Magnesium deficiency has also been seen in women suffering from PMS; medical studies have found a reduction in red blood cell magnesium during the second half of the menstrual cycle in affected women. Magnesium, like vitamin B6, is needed for the production of the beneficial prostaglandin hormones as well as for glucose metabolism. Magnesium supplements can also benefit women with severe emotionally triggered anxiety and insomnia. When taken before bedtime, magnesium helps to calm the mood and induce restful sleep.

Good food sources of magnesium include green leafy vegetables, beans and peas, raw nuts and seeds, tofu, avocados, raisins, dried figs, and millet and other grains. If you want to take magnesium as a supplement, I recommend increasing your magnesium supplement level to between 400-600 mg per day (reduce the dosage if it causes loose bowel movements or on your doctor's advice for other health conditions) or you can take liquid magnesium before bedtime, held under the tongue for two minutes.

*Potassium.* Like magnesium, potassium has a powerful enhancing effect on energy and vitality. Potassium deficiency has been associated with fatigue and muscular weakness, which is aggravated by anxiety and stress. One study showed that older people who were deficient in potassium had weaker grip strength. Potassium aspartate has been used with magnesium aspartate in a number of studies on chronic fatigue; this combination significantly restored energy levels.

Potassium has many important roles in the body. It constitutes 5 percent of the total mineral content of the body. It regulates the transfer of nutrients into the cells and works with sodium to maintain the body's water balance.

Its role in water balance is important in preventing PMS bloating symptoms. Potassium aids proper muscle contraction and transmission of electrochemical impulses. It helps maintain nervous system function and a healthy heart rate.

Potassium is commonly lost through chronic diarrhea or the excessive use of diuretics (which many women with PMS use to combat bloating around the time of their periods). In addition, the excessive use of coffee and alcohol (both of which can worsen anxiety and emotional stress symptoms) increases the loss of potassium through the urinary tract.

For women suffering from potassium loss, the use of a potassium supplement may be helpful. The most common dose available is a 99 mg tablet or capsule. I generally recommend one to three per day to be used up to one week before menstruation.

Potassium supplements, however, should be used cautiously in some women. They should be avoided if you have kidney or cardiovascular disease since a high level of potassium can cause an irregular heartbeat. Potassium also can be irritating to the intestinal tract, so it should be taken with meals. If you have any questions about the proper use of this mineral, ask your health-care provider. Happily, it is easy to take in sufficient levels of potassium from the diet. Potassium occurs in abundance in many fruits, vegetables, beans and peas, seeds and nuts, starches, and whole grains.

*Calcium.* Calcium is the most abundant mineral in the body. This important mineral helps combat stress, nervous tension, and anxiety. A calcium deficiency not only increases emotional irritability but also muscular irritability and cramps. Calcium can be taken at night along with magnesium to calm the mood and induce a restful sleep. This is particularly helpful for women with menopause-related anxiety, mood swings, and insomnia. Because calcium is a major structural component of bone, it has the added benefit of helping prevent bone loss, or osteoporosis.

Like magnesium and potassium, calcium is essential in the maintenance of regular heartbeat and the healthy transmission of impulses through the nerves. It may also help reduce blood pressure and regulate cholesterol levels; it is essential for blood clotting.

Many women do not take in the recommended daily allowance for calcium in their diet (800 mg for women during active reproductive years, 1000 to 1200 mg after menopause). In fact, many women take in only half the recommended amount. Good sources of calcium include green leafy vegetables, salmon (with bones), nuts and seeds, tofu, and blackstrap molasses. In addition, a calcium supplement may be useful.

*Zinc.* This mineral helps decrease anxiety and stress by facilitating the action of B vitamins, creating proper blood sugar balance as well as healthy immune function, digestion, and metabolism. Zinc is an essential trace mineral necessary for the absorption and action of vitamins, especially the anxiety and stress combating B vitamins. It is a constituent of many enzymes involved in metabolism and digestion.

Zinc helps reduce the anxiety due to blood sugar imbalances since it plays a role in normal carbohydrate digestion. It is a component of insulin, the protein that helps move glucose out of the blood circulation and into the cells. Once inside the cells, glucose provides them with their main source of energy.

In addition, zinc is part of the enzyme that is needed to break down alcohol. It is also necessary for the proper growth and development of the female reproductive tract and for effective wound healing. Zinc enhances the immune function, acting as an immune stimulant (it has been shown to trigger the reproduction of lymphocytes when incubated with these cells in a test tube).

Finally, zinc is needed for the synthesis of nucleic acids, which control the production of the different proteins in the body. Good food sources of zinc include wheat germ, pumpkin seeds, whole grain products, wheat bran, and high-protein foods. I recommend 15 – 25 mg of zinc per day taken as a supplement.

*Chromium and Manganese.* These two minerals are important in carbohydrate production and metabolism. Chromium helps keep the blood sugar level in balance by enhancing insulin function so glucose is properly utilized by the body. This prevents the extremes of too little glucose in the blood (hypoglycemia) or too much glucose (diabetes mellitus). By improving the intake of glucose into the cells, chromium helps the cells produce energy. Chromium accomplishes these functions through its participation in an important molecule called the glucose tolerance factor (GTF).

GTF is composed of chromium, niacin (vitamin B3), and three amino acids—glycerin, cysteine, and glutamic acid. This combination allows chromium to be available in the body in a biologically active form. Good sources of chromium include brewer's yeast, whole wheat, rye, oysters, potatoes, apples, bananas, spinach, molasses, and chicken. I recommend 150 mcg per day of chromium taken as a supplement.

Manganese aids glucose metabolism by acting as a cofactor in the process of converting glucose (food) to energy. It is also important in the digestion of food, especially proteins, and in the production of cholesterol and fatty acids in the body. Manganese is also needed for healthy bone growth and development as well as the production of the thyroid hormone, thyroxin. Food sources of manganese include nuts and whole grains. Seeds, beans, peas, and leafy green vegetables are also good sources when they have been grown in soil containing manganese. Animal foods tend to be low in this essential nutrient. An optimal dosage of manganese is 2 to 5 mg per day.

## Herbal Relief for Conditions Related To Anxiety

Many herbs can help to relieve the symptoms of anxiety and stress. I have used anxiety- and stress-relieving herbs in my practice for many years and many of my patients have found them to be effective remedies. Certain herbs can relax tension, ease anxiety and even promote restful sleep. Other herbs have mild immune-boosting and hormonal properties. They support the endocrine and the immune systems with a minimum of side effects. In this section, I describe many beneficial herbs that are useful for the relief of anxiety and stress-related symptoms.

### Herbs to Lower Cortisol and Boost Adrenals

Your adrenal glands produce the stress hormone cortisol. When you are under extreme, chronic stress, your body pours out continual amounts of cortisol. Over time, this excess cortisol can lead to fatigue, weight gain, insomnia, low immune function, and even premature aging. In contrast, low levels of cortisol can indicate that your adrenal glands have become exhausted and are not functioning properly.

Fortunately, DHEA balances the effects of cortisol. In this way, DHEA helps you better deal with all forms of stress, be it physical, mental, or emotional. To this end, many herbs have been shown to improve DHEA levels by helping to lower cortisol and boost adrenal function. I have used these herbs—namely rhodiola rosea, panax ginseng, Siberian ginseng, and licorice root—as well as the vitamin PABA in my practice for many years, and many of my patients have found them to be effective remedies.

**Rhodiola rosea** has been used medicinally for nearly 2,000 years. The ancient Greeks revered this rose-like rootstock, as did Siberian healers, who believed that people who drank Rhodiola tea on a regular basis would live to be more than 100 years old.

Rhodiola works to support all hormone production by easing stress and fatigue, both killers of adrenal function and healthy sex hormone production, including DHEA. According to the journal *Phytomedicine*, Rhodiola is particularly effective in fighting stress-induced fatigue. In one study, researchers tested 40 male medical students during exam time to determine if the herb positively affected physical fitness, as well as mental well-being and capacity. The students were divided into two groups and given either 50 mg of Rhodiola rosea extract or a placebo twice a day for 20 days. Researchers found that those students who took the extract had a significant decrease in mental fatigue and improved psychomotor function, with a 50 percent improvement in neuromotor function. Plus, scores from exams taken immediately after the study showed that the extract group had an average grade of 3.47, as compared to 3.20 for the placebo group.

To ease fatigue, stress, or anxiety—all of which can play havoc with your DHEA production—I recommend taking 50–100 mg of Rhodiola rosea three times a day, standardized to 3 percent rosavins and 0.8 percent salidrosides. While the herb is generally considered safe, some reports have indicated that it may counteract the effects of antiarrhythmic medications. Therefore, if you are currently taking this type of medication, I suggest you discuss the use of Rhodiola rosea with your physician.

**Panax ginseng** is an ivy-like ground cover originating in the wild, damp woodlands of northern China and Korea. Its use in Chinese herbal medicine dates back more than 4,000 years. In colonial North America, ginseng was a major export product. The wild form is now rare, but panax ginseng is a widely cultivated plant.

Ginseng has a legendary status among herbs. While extravagant claims have been made about its many uses, scientific research has yielded inconsistent results in verifying its therapeutic properties. However, enough good research does exist to demonstrate ginseng's activity, especially when high-quality extracts, standardized for active components, are used.

Ginseng has a balancing, tonic effect on the systems and organs of the body involved in the stress response. It contains at least 13 different saponins, a class of chemicals found in many plants, especially legumes, which take their name from their ability to form a soap-like froth when shaken with water. These compounds (triterpene glycosides) are the most pharmaceutically active constituents of ginseng. Saponins benefit hormone production, as well as cardiovascular function, immunity, and the central nervous system.

During times of stress and increased anxiety, the saponins in the ginseng act on the hypothalamus and pituitary glands, increasing the release of adrenocorticotrophin, or ACTH (a hormone produced by the pituitary that promotes the manufacture and secretion of adrenal hormones). As a result, ginseng increases the release of adrenal cortisone and other adrenal hormones, and prevents their depletion from stress.

Other substances associated with the pituitary are also released, such as endorphins. Ginseng is used to prevent adrenal atrophy, which can be a side effect of cortisone drug treatment. Ginseng's ability to support the health and function of the adrenal glands during times of stress, as well as the improved hormone health that occurs with the use of ginseng, clearly supports the production of DHEA itself by the adrenal glands.

In a double-blind study published in *Drugs Under Experimental and Clinical Research*, two groups of volunteers suffering from fatigue due to physical or mental stress were given nutritional supplementation over a 12-week period. One hundred sixty-three volunteers were given a multivitamin and multimineral complex, and 338 volunteers received the same product, plus a standardized Chinese ginseng extract. Once a month, the volunteers were asked to fill out a questionnaire during a scheduled visit with a physician. This questionnaire contained eleven questions that asked them to describe their current level of perceived physical energy, stamina, sense of well-being, libido, and quality of sleep.

While both groups experienced similar improvement in their quality of life by the second visit, the group using the ginseng extract almost doubled their improvement, based on their questionnaire responses, by the third and fourth visits. Thus, ginseng, when added to a multivitamin and multimineral complex, appears to improve many parameters of well-being in individuals experiencing significant physical and emotional stress.

There is also evidence that ACTH (the hormone that stimulates the adrenal cortex) and adrenal hormones, which ginseng stimulates, are known to bind to brain tissue, increasing mental activity during times of stress.

For maximum benefit, take a high-quality preparation, an extract of the main root of a plant that is six to eight years old, standardized for ginsenoside content and ratio. Companies manufacturing ginseng products may mention the age of the plants used in their products as a testimony to their products' quality. Take a 100 mg capsule twice a day. If this is too stimulating, especially before bedtime, take the second dose mid-afternoon, or take only the morning dose.

Women should avoid Korean red ginseng which has a heating and contracting effect on the body and can worsen anxiety and stress. Instead, use American or Chinese ginseng which has a more calming and cooling effect on the body and is beneficial if you are suffering from anxiety.

**Siberian ginseng** (Eleutherococcus senticosus) has been used in Asia for nearly 2,000 years to combat fatigue and increase endurance. The medicinal properties of this plant have been studied in Russia, with a number of clinical and experimental studies demonstrating that eleutherosides are adaptogenic, increasing resistance to stress and fatigue.

According to a review of clinical trials of more than 2,100 healthy human subjects, ranging in age from 19 to 72, published in *Economic Medicinal Plant Research*, Siberian ginseng reduces activation of the adrenal cortex in response to stress, an action useful in the alarm stage of the fight-or-flight response. It also helps lower blood pressure. In this same study, data indicated that the eleutherosides increased the subjects' ability to withstand adverse physical conditions including heat, noise, motion, an increase in workload, and exercise. There was also improved quality of work under stressful work conditions and improved athletic performance.

Herbalists have also long prescribed Siberian ginseng for chronic fatigue syndrome. One way in which ginseng may be effective in this capacity is through its ability to facilitate the conversion of fat into energy, in both intense and moderate physical activity, sparing carbohydrates, and postponing the point at which a person may "hit the wall." This occurs when stored glucose is depleted and can no longer serve as a source of energy.

Siberian ginseng is also used to treat a variety of psychological disturbances, including insomnia, hypochondriasis, and various neuroses. The reason this type of ginseng is effective may be its ability to balance stress hormones and neurotransmitters such as epinephrine, serotonin, and dopamine, all of which supports healthy hormone production, including DHEA and also reduce stress related symptoms.

Though Siberian ginseng has virtually no toxicity, individuals with fever, hypertonic crisis, or myocardial infarction are advised not to use it. A standard dosage of the dry powdered extract (containing at least one percent eleutheroside F) is 100–200 mg two times a day, taken in the morning and afternoon.

**Licorice root** has been enjoyed over the centuries as a sweet flavoring for candy and as a delicious tea, but it is also has powerful medicinal properties. Its medicinal use has been recorded historically for over 4,000 years. Respected by the ancient Egyptians, licorice was among the treasured items archaeologists discovered (in great quantities) when they opened King Tut's tomb. Sometime around the year 1600, John Josselyn of Boston listed licorice as one of the "precious herbs" brought from England to colonial America.

Licorice is used to treat respiratory conditions, urinary and kidney problems, fatty liver, hepatitis, the inflammation of arthritis, and ulcers. The herb also exhibits hormone-like activity. Licorice root increases the half-life of cortisol (the adrenal stress hormone), inhibiting the breakdown of adrenal hormones by the liver. As a result, licorice is useful in reversing low cortisol conditions, and in helping the adrenal glands rest and restore their function. This can help to improve our ability to handle stress and can reduce our level of anxiety.

A standard dosage is 1 to 2 g of powdered root or 450 to 600 mg in capsule form up to three times a day with meals. Licorice has activity similar to aldosterone, the adrenal hormone responsible for regulating water and electrolytes within the body. As a result, taking large doses of licorice (10 to 14 g of the crude herb) can lead to high blood pressure, water retention, and sodium and potassium imbalances. Licorice should not be taken by children under age two. Caution should also be used with older children, people over 65, nursing and pregnant women. Start with low dosages and increase the strength only if necessary.

## Herbs for Anxiety

**Sedative and Relaxant Herbs.** Kava root has been used for centuries in the Pacific islands to encourage a greater sense of well-being and relaxation during ceremonial events. Kava is currently being used to relieve symptoms of anxiety, stress, restlessness and insomnia. These benefits have been confirmed by clinical studies. The recommended dosage is 140 mg to 210 mg, either one hour before bedtime or three times a day for relief of anxiety and tension. One caution with using kava is that it has been linked to rare cases of liver damage. Do not use kava longer than four to eight weeks without consulting a physician.

Herbs such as valerian root, passionflower, hops, chamomile, and skullcap have a significant calming and restful effect on the central nervous system. With their mild sedative effect, they also promote restful sleep, a state that is difficult to induce when a woman is suffering from excessive anxiety and stress. Valerian root has been used extensively in traditional herbal medicine as a sleep inducer and is widely used both in Europe and the United States as a gentle herbal remedy to help combat insomnia. Valerian has an unpleasant taste, making it more palatable when taken in capsule form.

I have also been very pleased with the benefits these herbs have brought to my patients suffering from menopause-related anxiety and insomnia. Many women with moderate to severe symptoms of hormonal deficiency wake up two to three times a night. If you suffer from menopause-related insomnia, you may need to make a sedative tea like chamomile fairly strong, using as many as two or three tea bags in a cup of water.

Many women with anxiety also suffer from tight, tense muscles in vulnerable areas of their bodies (neck, shoulders, jaw, and the upper and lower back are common areas to store tension). Many of these relaxant herbs help to relieve the muscle tension and spasm that often accompany stress. Certain herbs like valerian root, peppermint, and chamomile are also effective in relieving stress-related indigestion and intestinal gas.

**Blood Circulation Enhancers.** Certain herbs such as ginger and ginkgo biloba improve circulation to the tight and tense muscles, thereby helping to relieve a common physiological response to anxiety. Ginger causes a widening or dilation of the blood vessels. Better blood circulation helps to draw nutrients to tight, tense muscles and also helps to remove waste products like lactic acid and carbon dioxide. As muscle metabolism improves, tension symptoms diminish. Ginger also has an antispasmodic effect on the smooth muscle of the intestinal tract and can help relieve digestive symptoms of excessive levels of anxiety and stress.

Besides taking ginger in tincture or capsule form, you can drink it as a delicious tea. To make ginger tea, buy a fresh ginger root at your super-market. Grate a few teaspoons of the fresh root into 4 cups of water. Boil gently and steep for 15-20 minutes. This is a very soothing herbal tea, delicious with a small amount of honey.

Ginkgo biloba also improves blood circulation and oxygenation to tense muscles. It has a vasodilating effect and decreases metabolic processes during a period of decreased blood supply. It is a very powerful herbal remedy and can be effectively combined with ginger.

## Herbs for Chronic Fatigue and Depression

Many women with anxiety also suffer from depression and fatigue. Anxiety and panic episodes can be exhausting to the body, stressing the endocrine and immune systems, and other important systems. Many women feel tired and depleted after anxiety episodes, since these episodes use up the body's available energy and nutrients. Women suffering from PMS, menopause, and hypoglycemia and food allergies can "roller coaster" between emotional highs and lows, even during a single day.

A number of herbs can help a woman experiencing excessive fatigue and depression alternating with anxiety due to anxiety episodes, PMS, and hypoglycemia. Herbs such as oat straw, ginger, ginkgo biloba, dandelion root, and Siberian ginseng (eleutherococcus) may have a stimulatory effect, improving energy and vitality. These herbs can improve one's ability to handle stress, as well as physical and mental energy.

St. John's wort is an herb that is currently used as a natural antidepressant and is being studied for its mood-altering effects. Extracts of St. John's wort, standardized to 0.3 hypericin (its active ingredient), have been found to have significant positive effects on depression without the negative side effects usually associated with prescription drugs. Use St. John's wort three times a day.

Siberian ginseng and ginger have been important traditional medicines in China and other countries for thousands of years. They have been reputed to increase longevity and decrease fatigue and weakness. In modern China, Japan, and other countries, there is a great deal of interest in the pharmacological effects of these traditional herbs. Scientific studies are corroborating the medicinal effects of these plants. These herbs boost immunity and strengthen the cardiovascular system. The bioflavonoids contained in ginkgo are extremely powerful antioxidants and help combat fatigue by improving circulation to the brain. They also appear to have a strong affinity for the adrenal and thyroid glands and may boost function in these essential glands.

### Herbs for Menopause and PMS

Many plants can be useful in the treatment of both PMS and menopause because they actually contain small amounts of the female hormones estrogen and progesterone. These plants, called phytoestrogens, include the following:

**Bioflavonoid-Containing Plants.** Bioflavonoids were also discussed in the vitamin section. In their purified form, they help to relieve symptoms of both estrogen imbalance and deficiency as well as heavy menstrual flow. However, some women may want to use the actual plant sources of the bioflavonoids as part of their nutritional program. This approach has some benefits because whole plant extracts often contain a wide range of useful nutrients that support the therapeutic effects of the bioflavonoids themselves. As mentioned earlier, bioflavonoids occur in a large variety of fruits and flowers. Excellent sources include citrus fruits, cherry, grape, and hawthorn berry. All of these plants are available in capsule or tincture form for women wanting to use them as herbal supplements.

Many medical studies of citrus bioflavonoids have demonstrated their usefulness in treating menopause-related hot flashes and insomnia. They are also useful in controlling menopause-related anxiety and mood swings because they have weak estrogenic activity (1/50,000 the strength of a drug dose of estrogen). Plants containing bioflavonoids may be especially useful for women who cannot or do not choose to use standard estrogen replacement therapy. This is often the case in women with pre-existing health problems like breast or uterine cancer, hypotension, or blood clots.

In addition, women who have already experienced side effects from estrogen such as bloating, breast tenderness, or even a worsening of anxiety symptoms or mood swings may not wish to continue on prescription estrogen. The very low potency of bioflavonoids make them ideal nutrients for menopause because the risk of side effects is minimal.

Because bioflavonoids are also antiestrogenic, herbs containing high levels of this nutrient are useful in stabilizing mood and reducing anxiety in my PMS patients. PMS mood symptoms can be linked in some women to an estrogen-progesterone imbalance. Both of these hormones affect brain chemistry and mood. Progesterone has a sedative-like effect while estrogen in excess can worsen anxiety symptoms. Thus, the proper balance between the two female hormones is quite important.

**Other Phytoestrogens.** Other phytoestrogen plant sources of estrogen and progesterone used in traditional herbal medicine for menopause symptoms include dong quai, black cohosh, blue cohosh, unicorn root, false unicorn root, fennel, anise, sarsaparilla, and wild yam root. The hormonal activities of these plants have been observed in a number of interesting research studies.

Plants may also form the basis for the production of medical hormones in the laboratory. Many common plants such as soybeans and wild yams contain a preformed steroidal nucleus. Estrogen and progesterone can be synthesized from plants in relatively few steps and have allowed prescription female sex hormones to become widely commercially available.

*Herbs for Food Allergies and Hypoglycemia*

Many herbs can be used to help the digestive process and stabilize the blood sugar level. Symptoms of digestive upset such as irritable bowel syndrome and reactions to eating various foods are commonly triggered by anxiety, stress and panic attacks. Blood sugar imbalances are also worsened by anxiety. Beneficial herbs to treat these issues include the following:

**Herbal Digestive Aids.** Many herbs reduce symptoms of food intolerance such as bloating, abdominal cramps, diarrhea, constipation, fatigue, headache, and mood swings by improving the digestive process. They do this by aiding in the more efficient breakdown of food to basic constituents (amino acids, fatty acids, simple sugars, etc.) and by improving the absorption and assimilation of foods.

Papaya leaf contains powerful enzymes — papain and chymopapain — that help digest protein. These enzymes promote food digestion in women with liver or pancreatic-related health problems. The enzymes in papaya leaf (or the whole papaya fruit itself) are an important ingredient in dozens of commercial digestive aids. Though papaya leaf has no direct effect on hypoglycemia, it does indirectly help stabilize the blood sugar level by helping break down complex protein- and carbohydrate-containing foods, making their nutrients more available.

Ginger also helps improve digestion and assimilation of foods from the digestive tract into the general circulation. It does this by promoting better blood circulation to the digestive tract, by relaxing smooth muscles in the intestines, and by stimulating the metabolism. Ginger also reduces symptoms of nausea. Like papaya leaf, it has an indirect effect on stabilizing the blood sugar level by helping to increase the availability of essential nutrients through more efficient digestive processes.

Peppermint and fennel also help to calm upset stomach, normalize bowel function, and eliminate heartburn and intestinal spasm. Peppermint also has anti-inflammatory and anti-infective properties that can help promote healthier intestinal absorption and assimilation. Peppermint (and other members of the mint family) has also been found in research studies to have potent antiviral, antibacterial, and antifungal effects. Garlic is another powerful herb that helps to normalize the digestive process by inhibiting pathological microorganisms such as fungi, viruses, and bacteria, and promoting the growth of beneficial flora. It is particularly useful in the suppression of intestinal candida. Overgrowth of a pathogenic fungus, candida albicans, can cause a variety of unpleasant digestive symptoms.

**Blood Sugar Stabilizers.** Several herbs have been found to stabilize the blood sugar level, thereby reducing the effect that anxiety and mood swings have on triggering symptoms of hypoglycemia.

Most prominent among these herbs is Siberian ginseng. This herb is an adaptogen, which helps to protect the body against the effects of both physical and mental stress. It has a normalizing effect on the blood sugar level, raising it when it falls too low and decreasing it when it becomes abnormally high.

Siberian ginseng also helps reduce anxiety and mood swings by its ability to improve adrenal function, thus protecting the body from the harmful effects of stress. The use of Siberian ginseng allows people to withstand increased workloads, exercise levels, and noise, among other stress factors. It also improves mental alertness and energy levels and helps decrease fatigue in women with anxiety symptoms. The effects of Siberian ginseng build up over time; therefore, you may need to use it for several weeks to months before experiencing symptom relief.

Gotu kola helps to stabilize the blood sugar level by improving adrenal function. It behaves similarly to Siberian ginseng, acting as a potent anti-fatigue nutrient. Women who are experiencing excessive levels of anxiety may find the energy-supporting qualities of both these herbs to be quite helpful during stressful periods.

## Essential Fatty Acids for Relief of Anxiety

Essential fatty acids are an extremely important part of the nutritional program for any women with anxiety and stress symptoms. Essential fatty acids must be taken in through the diet and are the raw materials from which the beneficial hormone-like chemicals called prostaglandins are made.

Beneficial series-1 and series-3 prostaglandins help to create mood and hormone balance within the body. They also have muscle relaxant and blood vessel relaxant properties that can significantly reduce your level of emotional tension and muscle cramps. They reduce inflammation within the body. Inflammatory conditions such as food allergies and autoimmune diseases are often aggravated by anxiety and stress.

Prostaglandins have a calming and relaxing effect on the emotions through their beneficial effect on the brain. Taking in sufficient essential fatty acids in the diet can reduce the severity of agitation, sleeplessness, depression and bipolar disorder. Because of their beneficial effects, they have been used in the treatment of PMS, anxiety, eating disorders, and menopause.

Essential fatty acids also help to balance your levels of female hormones and are needed for the production of progesterone during the second half of the menstrual cycle. Progesterone counters the mood elevating and anxiety producing effects of estrogen with its calming and sedative effects. Adequate production of progesterone and even treatment with bioidentical progesterone is very important if you suffer from anxiety and panic attacks. I discuss bioidentical progesterone in the chapter on drug therapies further on in this book.

There are two main essential types of essential fatty acids that are extremely beneficial for women and help to reduce your vulnerability to anxiety and stress. These are linoleic acid, which belongs to the omega-6 family of fatty acids, and is primarily found in raw seeds and nuts. Good sources include flaxseed, pumpkin seeds, sesame seeds, sunflower seeds and walnuts. Omega-6 fatty acids are converted into the series-1 prostaglandins.

The omega-3 family of essential fatty acids are derived from both animal and plant sources in our diet. These include EPA (eicosapentaenoic acid) and DHA (docosahexaenoic acid) that are found in certain fish such as trout, salmon, tuna and mackerel. Alpha-linolenic acid is a member of the omega-3 family as well and found in plant sources like flaxseeds, chia seeds, hemp seed oil, and in smaller amounts, in soy, pumpkin seeds, walnuts and green leafy vegetables. The omega-3 fatty acids are converted into the beneficial series-3 prostaglandins within the body.

Both essential fatty acid families must be derived from dietary sources because they cannot be produced within the body. However, even if the diet contains significant amounts of fatty acids, some women may lack the ability to convert them efficiently to the mood and hormone balancing prostaglandins. This is particularly true of linoleic acid, which must be converted to a chemical called gamma-linolenic acid (GLA) on its way to becoming the beneficial series-1 prostaglandin.

The conversion of linoleic acid to GLA, followed by the chemical steps leading to the creation of the beneficial prostaglandins, requires the presence of magnesium, vitamin B6, zinc, vitamin C, and niacin. Women deficient in these nutrients can't make the chemical conversions effectively. These nutrients are also needed for the conversion of the omega-3 fatty acids into the series-3 prostaglandins.

In addition, women who eat a high cholesterol diet, eat processed oils such as mayonnaise, use a great deal of alcohol, or are diabetic may find the fatty acid conversion to the series-1 prostaglandin difficult to achieve. Other factors that impede prostaglandin production include emotional stress, allergies, and eczema. In women with these risk factors, less than 1 percent of linoleic acid may be converted to GLA. The rest of the fatty acids may be used as an energy source, but they will not be able to play a role in relieving anxiety and stress symptoms.

The best plant food sources of the omega-3 essential fatty acids are raw flaxseeds and chia seeds, which contain high levels of both essential fatty acids, alpha-linolenic and linoleic acid. Both the seeds and their pressed oils can be used and should be absolutely fresh and unspoiled. As mentioned earlier, these oils become rancid very easily when exposed to light and air (oxygen), and they need to be packed in special opaque containers and kept in the refrigerator.

My special favorite is fresh flaxseed oil; golden, rich and delicious. It is extremely high in alpha-linolenic and linoleic acids, which comprise approximately 80 percent of its total content. Flax oil has a wonderful flavor and can be used as a butter replacement on foods such as mashed potatoes, rice, air-popped popcorn, steamed broccoli, cauliflower, carrots and bread. Flax oil (and all other essential oils) should never be heated or used in cooking, as heat affects the special chemical properties of these oils. Instead, add these oils as a flavoring to foods that are already cooked.

Chia seeds are very nutritious edible seeds that were a staple of the Aztec diet. Like flaxseeds, they are loaded with beneficial omega-3 fatty acids as well as protein and fiber. Because they are a rich source of alpha-linolenic acid, they can be very beneficial in the treatment of PMS and menopause that commonly cause mood symptoms and anxiety.

Chia seeds also have other health benefits. Because omega-3's are anti-inflammatory, they help to reduce "false fat" and bloating. They provide relief from other inflammatory conditions including allergies, sinusitis, bronchitis, colds and autoimmune diseases like rheumatoid arthritis and lupus. They also help to regulate your blood sugar level and control diabetes as well as reduce your risk of heart disease

You can eat up to one ounce of chia seeds a day. I recommend sprinkling it into yogurt, oatmeal, smoothies, applesauce or salad or even mix it into your pancake, waffle mix, or flour for baking.

EPA and DHA (omega-3 family) are found in abundance in fish oils. The best sources are cold-water, high-fat fish such as salmon, tuna, rainbow trout, mackerel, and eel. Fish can be used in your diet once or twice a week but more frequent use of fish should be limited because of the high levels of mercury found in many fish.

Instead, I recommend using mercury-free fish oil capsules as a daily supplement. You should use fish oil supplements, which contain 2000-3000 mg of eicosapentaenoic acid (EPA) and docosa-hexaenoic acid (DHA). Vegetarians can use algae (seaweed) supplements of DHA and EPA.

Linoleic acid (omega-6 family) is found in many seeds and seed oils. Good sources include safflower oil, sunflower oil, corn oil, sesame seed oil, and wheat germ oil. Many women prefer to use fresh raw sesame seeds, sunflower seeds, and wheat germ to obtain the oils.

The average healthy adult requires only four teaspoons per day of the essential oils. However, women with anxiety and stress symptoms who may have a real deficiency of these oils need up to two tablespoons per day until their symptoms improve. Occasionally, these oils may cause diarrhea; if this occurs, use only one teaspoon per day. Women with acne and very oily skin should use them cautiously. For optimal results, be sure to use these oils along with vitamin E.

## Nutritional Supplements for Women with Anxiety and Stress

Good dietary habits are crucial for control of your anxiety and stress symptoms. But for many women, the use of nutritional supplements is important in order to achieve high levels of the essential nutrients needed to heal anxiety and stress. On the following pages is a sample of the vitamins and minerals as well as their dosages that can be used as a foundation for your program. You can also add the other nutrients like flaxseed oil and fish oil that I have discussed in this chapter to fill out your program.

You may find it easier to implement your program if you start with one of the better quality multinutrient products for women that are available in health food stores and through the Internet and then add the remaining essential nutrients.

Remember that all women differ somewhat in their nutritional needs. If you do take the recommended vitamin or herbal supplements, I usually advise that you start with one-fourth to one-half the dose recommended in this book and work your way up slowly to the higher dosage, if needed. You may find that you do best with slightly more or less of certain ingredients.

I recommend that patients take their supplements with meals or at least a snack. Very rarely, a woman will have a digestive reaction to supplements, such as nausea or indigestion. If this happens, stop all supplements; then resume using them, adding one at a time, until you find the offending nutrient. Eliminate from your program any nutrient to which you have a reaction. If you have any specific questions, ask a health care professional who is knowledgeable about nutrition.

## Summary Chart For Nutritional Supplements

I want to end this section by summarizing the nutritional supplements that you can take to help eliminate your anxiety symptoms. These include:

1. **Vitamins, Minerals and Phytoestrogens** - Vitamin B-Complex, Vitamin C, Soy Isoflavones, Bioflavonoids, Vitamin E, Magnesium, Potassium, Zinc, Calcium, Chromium and Manganese.

2. **Essential Fatty Acids** -

> *Omega-6 fatty acids*: evening primrose oil, borage oil, black currant oil, pumpkin seeds, sesame seeds, sunflower seeds and walnuts.

> *Omega-3 fatty acids*: flaxseeds, chia seeds, hempseed and EPA and DHA-rich fish such as salmon, tuna, rainbow trout, mackerel, and halibut.

3. **Amino Acids** – 5-HTP (5-hydroxytryptophan), GABA (gamma amino butric acid), tyrosine, taurine, L-theanine, melatonin.

## Summary Chart of Herbs

|  | Herbs |
|---|---|
| **Herbs to Lower Cortisol and Boost Adrenals** | Rhodiola rosea<br>Panax ginseng<br>Siberian ginseng<br>Licorice root |
| **Sedative and Relaxant Herbs** | Kava root<br>Valerian root<br>Passionflower<br>Celery hops<br>Chamomile<br>Skullcap<br>Balm Bay<br>Motherwort |
| **Blood Circulation Enhancers** | Ginger<br>Ginkgo biloba |
| **Herbs for Chronic Fatigue and Depression** | Oat straw<br>Ginger<br>Ginkgo biloba<br>Dandelion root<br>Siberian ginseng<br>St. John's wort |
| **Herbs for Menopause and PMS** | Dong quai<br>Black cohosh<br>Blue cohosh<br>Unicorn root<br>Fennel<br>Anise<br>Sarsaparilla<br>Wild yam root<br>Citrus fruit rind and pulp<br>Red clover |
| **Herbal Digestive Aids** | Fennel<br>Garlic<br>Ginger<br>Peppermint |
| **Blood Sugar Stabilizers** | Siberian ginseng<br>Gotu kola |

## Optimal Nutritional Supplement Formula for Anxiety and Stress

Vitamins and Minerals
| | |
|---|---|
| Vitamin A | 5000 I.U. |
| Beta-Carotene (provitamin A) | 25,000 I.U. |
| Vitamin B-Complex | |
|   B1 (thiamine) | 50-100 mg |
|   B2 (riboflavin) | 50-100 mg |
|   B3 (niacinamide) | 50-100 mg |
|   B5 (pantothenic acid) | 50-200 mg |
|   B6 (pyridoxine) | 50-100 mg |
|   B12 (cyanocobalamin) | 100-750 mcg |
|   Folic acid | 400-800 mcg |
|   Biotin | 400 mcg |
|   Choline | 250-500 mg |
|   Inositol | 250-500 mg |
|   PABA (para-aminobenzoic acid) | 50-100 mg |
| Vitamin C (as mineral ascorbates) | 2000-5000 mg |
| Vitamin D | 1000 I.U. |
| Vitamin E (d-alpha tocopherol acetate) | 400-800 I.U. |
| Calcium | 500-1000 mg |
| Magnesium | 250-500 mg |
| Potassium | 100-200 mg |
| Iron | 18 mg |
| Chromium | 150 mcg |
| Manganese | 5 mg |
| Selenium | 200 mcg |
| Zinc | 15 mg |
| Copper | 2 mg |
| Iodine | 150 mcg |

Dosage: Take one-quarter to the full amount of the above nutrients on a daily basis. Begin this formula with the lowest dose of each nutrient and increase the dose slowly and gradually to the recommended maximum, depending on how you are feeling.

## Food Sources of Vitamin A

**Vegetables**
Carrots
Carrot juice
Collard greens
Dandelion greens
Green onions
Kale
Parsley
Spinach
Sweet potatoes
Turnip greens
Winter squash

**Fruits**
Apricots
Avocado
Cantaloupe
Mangoes
Papaya
Peaches
Persimmons

**Meat, poultry, seafood**
Crab
Halibut
Liver—all types
Mackerel
Salmon
Swordfish

## Food Sources of Vitamin B-Complex (including folic acid)

**Vegetables**
Alfalfa
Artichoke
Asparagus
Beets
Broccoli
Brussels sprouts
Cabbage
Cauliflower
Green beans
Kale
Leeks
Onions
Peas
Romaine lettuce

**Legumes**
Garbanzo beans
Lentils
Lima beans
Pinto beans
Soybeans

**Meat, poultry, seafood**
Egg yolks*
Liver*

**Grains**
Barley
Bran
Brown rice
Corn Millet
Rice bran
Wheat
Wheat germ

**Sweeteners**
Blackstrap molasses

*Eggs and meat should be from organic, range-free stock fed on pesticide-free food.*

## Food Sources of Vitamin B6

| Grains | Vegetables | Meat, poultry, seafood |
|---|---|---|
| Brown rice | Asparagus | Chicken |
| Buckwheat flour | Beet greens | Salmon |
| Rice bran | Broccoli | Shrimp |
| Rye flour | Brussels sprouts | Tuna |
| Wheat germ | Cauliflower | |
| Whole wheat flour | Green peas | **Nuts and seeds** |
| | Leeks | Sunflower seeds |
| | Sweet potatoes | |

## Food Sources of Vitamin C

| Fruits | Vegetables and legumes | Meat, poultry, seafood |
|---|---|---|
| Blackberries | Asparagus | Liver—all types |
| Black currants | Black-eyed peas | Pheasant |
| Cantaloupe | Broccoli | Quail |
| Elderberries | Brussels sprouts | Salmon |
| Grapefruit | Cabbage | |
| Grapefruit juice | Cauliflower | |
| Guavas | Collards | |
| Kiwi fruit | Green onions | |
| Mangoes | Green peas | |
| Oranges | Kale | |
| Orange juice | Kohlrabi | |
| Pineapple | Parsley | |
| Raspberries | Potatoes | |
| Strawberries | Rutabagas | |
| Tangerines | Sweet pepper | |
| Tomatoes | Sweet potatoes | |
| | Turnips | |

## Food Sources of Vitamin E

**Vegetables**
Asparagus
Cucumber
Green peas
Kale

**Nuts and seeds**
Almonds
Brazil nuts
Hazelnuts
Peanuts

**Meats, poultry, seafood**
Haddock
Herring
Mackerel
Lamb
Liver — all types

**Oils**
Corn
Peanut
Safflower
Sesame
Soybean
Wheat germ

**Grains**
Brown rice
Millet

**Fruits**
Mangoes

## Food Sources of Essential Fatty Acids

**Oils**
Flax
Pumpkin
Soybean
Walnut
Safflower

Sunflower
Grape
Corn
Wheat germ
Sesame

## Food Sources of Iron

### Grains
Bran cereal (All-Bran)
Bran muffin
Millet, dry
Oat flakes
Pasta, whole wheat
Pumpernickel bread
Wheat germ

### Legumes
Black beans
Black-eyed peas
Garbanzo beans
Kidney beans
Lentils
Lima beans
Pinto beans
Soybeans
Split peas
Tofu

### Vegetables
Beets
Beet greens
Broccoli
Brussels sprouts
Corn
Dandelion greens
Green beans
Kale
Leeks
Spinach
Sweet potatoes
Swiss chard

### Fruits
Apple juice
Avocado
Blackberries
Dates, dried
Figs
Prunes, dried
Prune juice
Raisins

### Meat, poultry, seafood
Beef liver
Calf's liver
Chicken liver
Clams
Oysters
Sardines
Scallops
Trout

### Nuts and seeds
Almonds
Pecans
Pistachios
Sesame butter
Sesame seeds
Sunflower seeds

# Food Sources of Calcium

**Vegetables and legumes**
Artichoke
Black beans
Black-eyed peas
Beet greens
Broccoli
Brussels sprouts
Cabbage
Collards
Eggplant
Garbanzo beans
Green beans
Green onions
Kale
Kidney beans
Leeks
Lentils
Parsley
Parsnips
Pinto beans
Rutabagas
Soybeans
Spinach
Turnips
Watercress

**Meat, poultry, seafood**
Abalone
Beef
Bluefish
Carp
Crab
Haddock
Herring
Lamb
Lobster
Oysters
Perch
Salmon
Shrimp
Venison

**Fruits**
Blackberries
Black currants
Boysenberries
Oranges
Pineapple juice
Prunes
Raisins
Rhubarb
Tangerine juice

**Grains**
Bran
Brown rice
Bulgar wheat
Millet

## Food Sources of Magnesium

**Vegetables and legumes**
Artichoke
Black-eyed peas
Carrot juice
Corn
Green peas
Leeks
Lima beans
Okra
Parsnips
Potatoes
Soybean sprouts
Spinach
Squash
Yams
Snapper
Turkey
Papaya

**Meat, poultry, seafood**
Beef
Carp
Chicken
Clams
Cod
Crab
Duck
Haddock
Herring
Lamb
Mackerel
Oysters
Salmon
Shrimp
Raisins
Prunes

**Nuts and seeds**
Almonds
Brazil nuts
Hazelnuts
Peanuts
Pistachios
Pumpkin seeds
Sesame seeds
Walnuts

**Fruits**
Avocado
Banana
Grapefruit juice
Pineapple juice

**Grains**
Millet
Brown rice
Wild rice

## Food Sources of Potassium

### Vegetables and legumes
Artichoke
Asparagus
Black-eyed peas
Beets
Brussels sprouts
Carrot juice
Cauliflower
Corn
Garbanzo beans
Green beans
Kidney beans
Leeks
Lentils
Lima beans
Navy beans
Okra
Parsnips
Peas
Pinto beans
Potatoes
Pumpkin
Soybean sprouts
Spinach
Squash
Yams

### Meat, poultry, seafood
Bass
Beef
Carp
Catfish
Chicken
Cod
Duck
Eel
Flatfish
Haddock
Halibut
Herring
Lamb
Lobster
Mackerel
Oysters
Perch
Pike
Salmon
Scallops
Shrimp
Snapper
Trout
Turkey
Raisins

### Nuts and seeds
Almonds
Brazil nuts
Chestnuts
Hazelnuts
Macadamia nuts
Peanuts
Pistachios
Pumpkin seeds
Sesame seeds
Sunflower seeds
Walnuts

### Fruits
Apricots
Avocado
Banana
Cantaloupe
Currants
Figs
Grapefruit juice
Orange juice
Papaya
Pineapple juice
Prunes

### Grains
Brown rice
Millet
Wild rice

## Food Sources of Zinc

### Grains
Barley
Brown rice
Buckwheat
Corn
Cornmeal
Millet
Oatmeal
Rice bran
Rye bread
Wheat bran
Wheat germ
Wheat berries
Whole wheat bread
Whole wheat flour

### Vegetables and Legumes
Black-eyed peas
Cabbage
Carrots
Garbanzo beans
Green peas
Lentils
Lettuce
Lima beans
Onions
Soy flour
Soy meal
Soy protein

### Fruits
Apples
Peaches

### Meat, Poultry, Seafood
Chicken
Oysters

# 8

# Renewing Your Mind with Love, Peace and Joy

This is one of my favorite chapters in the book because I share with you many wonderful meditations and exercises that you can use to repattern your mind and emotions away from anxiety and stress towards a greater sense of love, peace and joy. Even if the cause of your anxiety is due to a physical illness, a positive, peaceful and relaxed mindset will help to improve your health by balancing your brain chemistry and hormones and supporting healthy immunity. You can use these meditations and exercises in addition to the psychological therapies offered by conventional medicine with great benefit.

Many doctors and psychologists recommend talk therapy and participating in support groups, along with medication, to help manage anxiety, panic attacks and stress. When engaging in talk therapy, you are consulting with mental health professionals in a calm and safe environment. It gives you the opportunity to discuss your feelings of anxiety or panic that can occur in response to life experiences such as phobias around attending social situations, dealing with difficult relationships, public speaking and even past traumas.

The goal is to learn how to work your way through these feelings and release the charge associated with the experiences that are stress inducing. You work towards desensitizing to the experiences so that, over time, they become less anxiety producing or traumatic. In the process, you also learn ways to change your behavior through better coping and communication skills.

Your therapist may also help you learn new and more effective ways to relax when experiencing stress. Some therapists let the client guide the therapeutic process, while acting as a sounding board or guide to the client's own innate healing process.

Some women find joining a support group of like-minded people who are also dealing with anxiety symptoms to be beneficial. In support groups, the members come together in a sharing and caring environment in which people can openly discuss their personal issues and look to other members of the group for positive support and possible solutions. A support group can be a great place to meet others who are struggling with similar issues.

While talk therapy and support groups can be very beneficial, there is also a great deal that you can do on your own to transform your emotions and repattern your feelings away from anxiety and stress towards relaxation, peace and joy.

In modern times, thousands of studies have been done that give scientific validity to the age-old wisdom that what you do with your mind and emotions has a powerful effect on your health. This is why I advocate focusing your time, attention, and energy on those positive emotions that build you up and enhance the quality of your life and your life force instead of spiraling you down into anxiety, stress and ill health. These include prayer, love, gratitude, appreciation, laughter and happiness, optimism, a positive self-image, and generosity.

Each of these positive practices and emotions helps to replace and eliminate anxiety and worry producing thoughts and beliefs so that you become a much more relaxed, calm and joyful person. In this chapter, I share with you many wonderful processes and exercises that you can use to build up and reinforce a strong emotional foundation of positive thoughts and feelings in your mind.

I recommend that you read through this chapter and try the exercises that appeal to you. If you practice them regularly, over time these positive beliefs and emotions will become your main point of focus when interfacing with the world around you.

## The Power of Prayer

One of my patients, Maria, shared her wonderful story with me about how prayer and her faith in God finally enabled her to heal from crippling anxiety and panic episodes. Several years ago, her anxiety was so severe that she could barely function. She avoided friends and almost became a shut-in because of the intensity of her symptoms.

Maria felt constantly overcome by fear and worry; she had difficulty falling asleep and staying asleep and would sometimes wake up in the middle of the night gasping for air with terrifying nightmares. She had episodes of feeling like her heart was racing, chest tightness, pain in her stomach, intestinal cramping and cold hands and feet. She consulted with psychiatrists, psychologist, did talk therapy and used medication but felt that nothing really helped.

A lapsed Christian who rarely attended church, she finally, in desperation, turned to God and got down on her knees and prayed for relief and healing. She said that she suddenly felt the presence of angels around her and heard a voice inside of her that she would be all right. To her amazement, her anxiety and panic episodes disappeared and she was healed. She said that she was totally transformed by this experience. Her great faith in and love for God has continued to this day. She prays everyday and feels immense gratitude for the healing that she received from our loving and merciful Creator.

Unfortunately, the great benefits of spiritual practices like prayer and the incredible role of God in promoting healing is mostly ignored in the field of medicine. I firmly believe that spirituality absolutely has a role in medicine and I have firsthand experienced the power of prayer with many of my patients, my friends and family as well as myself. I want to share with you several other very inspirational stories of the power of prayer.

## Michael's Story

When I first saw Michael, he was in the ICU of the hospital on life support. He had suffered a bleeding episode in his brain and was in very serious condition.

Although his family was living outside of the country, he was blessed by having a large number of devoted friends who constantly visited him and watched over him. Yet, despite being given the best medical care, he continued to be in a very fragile state and remained unconscious.

His doctors finally felt that he had no chance for recovery and were seriously considering taking him off life support. We prayed very hard for a miracle to occur and the next day I received a very excited call from his best friend telling me that Michael had opened his eyes. I rushed over to the hospital and found that not only were his eyes open but he gave me the thumbs up sign as I was leaving his room.

His recovery went very fast from that time on. Even his doctor said that he considered Michael's recovery a true miracle. Michael told me that he remembered all of us praying for him, even though he was unconscious. Tears of gratitude rolled down his face as he expressed his appreciation for our prayers and to God for saving his life and giving him another chance to be with his loved ones, friends and family.

## Alicia's Story

I am always inspired by the power of prayer and love! Recently, I was at the hospital visiting with a woman, Alicia, who had been in a car accident. She had broken her pelvic bones and had injuries to her chest and back. Alicia was in extreme pain, which became worse if she even tried to adjust her position. She was also on oxygen therapy to help her breathe.

Alicia was scheduled for surgery the next day to stabilize her fractured bones, which would greatly lengthen her recovery time. I visited her quite a bit and we prayed together several times. Each time we prayed together, she said that her level of pain diminished.

When I next saw her, I was thrilled to find Alicia lying in bed with a huge smile, surrounded by balloons and flowers and lots of visitors. She had a large family who lived locally and they were all gathered around her and were handling all of the paper work and other details from the hospital. She felt totally loved and nurtured by all of this positive support and attention.

Alicia's recovery was also improving rapidly. Her level of pain had greatly decreased; she was off the oxygen therapy and was breathing much better. Best of all, her doctors had cancelled the surgery, deciding that she could recover very well on supportive care and rehabilitation. She shared with me that she was thrilled to be feeling so much better and felt that the tide had turned with all of the prayers along with the loving and positive support of her family!

### Research Confirms the Power of Prayer

Studies from around the world are also confirming the healing power of prayer. One study looked at the cardiac care unit of a hospital in the San Francisco area. Researchers divided the patients into two groups. The patients in the first group were prayed for and those in the second group were not. Researchers found that those people who had prayers said for them had less risk of congestive heart failure and cardiac arrest, and fewer of them needed diuretics and antibiotics, as compared to the group that was not prayed for.

Similarly, a group of 40 AIDS patients were divided into two groups—one that was prayed for 6 days a week for 10 weeks and one that was not prayed for at all. Again, researchers found that the prayed-for group did considerably better than the others. They had significantly fewer new AIDS-related illnesses, saw their physicians less often, and spent less time in the hospital.

In a study reported in the *Journal of Reproductive Medicine*, researchers tested nearly 200 women who were undergoing in vitro fertilization at a clinic in Seoul, Korea. All were of similar age and had similar fertility concerns. They were divided into two groups. Several prayer groups from the U.S., Canada, and Australia were given photographs of the women in the first group and prayed for the women for four months. Neither the women nor the researchers knew who was being prayed for and who wasn't. At the end of the four months, twice as many women who were prayed for became pregnant as compared to the women in the control group.

In a similar double-blind, placebo-controlled study published in the *American Heart Journal*, researchers divided 150 heart patients (all of whom were scheduled for angioplasty) into five groups. One group received guided imagery therapy, the second had stress relaxation, the third had healing touch, the fourth were prayed for, and the last received no complementary therapy. Neither the patients, physicians, staff, nor family members knew which patients were being prayed for. After the procedures, those patients who were prayed for had fewer complications than patients in any of the other groups. Researchers were so amazed at the outcome that they have since enrolled over 300 more people for additional studies.

According to a *USA Weekend* poll, more than 75 percent of adults believe that spirituality and prayer can help you recover from an illness or injury, with 56 percent of these same adults saying that they personally have been helped by faith and prayer. And when asked how they felt about having their doctor discuss spirituality, nearly two-thirds felt that it would be a good idea.

But given all this, the reality is that only 10 percent of physicians address spiritual beliefs and needs with their patients. It would be much better to acknowledge the spiritual needs and concerns of our patients to support their healing from illness. As a physician, I have found that asking patients about their faith helps me understand any emotional and spiritual blocks that might be contributing to their condition and support my patients in their faith. I am also able to learn more about the patients' support network, which helps me to ensure that they have the type of care that will enable them to heal and resume living a full and vital life.

I wrote these spiritually inspired meditations and want to share them with you to support your emotional and mental transformation from fear, worry and anxiety to faith, hope, peace, joy and inner strength and reinforce your connection to the Divine source of life and goodness.

- May love, kindness, and compassion fill your heart each day. May you recognize the light of God in everyone close to you and in everyone you encounter in life's journey. May love, kindness, and compassion soften and illuminate your heart, casting a warm glow on the world around you.

- During difficult times, it is important to draw upon your inner strength to help you successfully meet the challenges in your life. Know that you can rely on your inner reserves of courage and self-confidence to help you make the right choices and decisions. At the same time, you need to be flexible in your approach, willing to change course, and allow yourself to find new and even better solutions when confronted with road blocks or challenges.

- Remember that each day is a fresh beginning. Your life, health, and sense of well-being benefits immeasurably when you live each day joyfully, filled with the positive expectations of the many good things that flow to you. It is with this positive attitude that you align yourself with Divine light and love.

I want to share with you one of my favorite meditations. It is a beautiful meditation on filling yourself with the Divine light and love of God. This meditation will also help you release any anxiety, tension or negativity from your mind and fill you with wonderful feelings of peace and joy.

- Begin the meditation by finding a quiet place. It can be a peaceful room in your house or office or even a beautiful spot in your backyard.

- Then, sit or lie in a comfortable position, with your arms resting gently by your sides.

- Close your eyes and breathe deeply. Let your breathing be slow and relaxed.

- Visualize yourself as a flower in the sun, opening yourself to God's light and love. Feel this Divine light surrounding you and enfolding you, filling every cell of your body with love.

- As this light fills and nurtures you, you are being cleansed of all cares and worries. This Divine light is dispelling all darkness as it gently and lovingly restores you to a state of health, balance and peace.

- Visualize this Divine light, bringing brightness and clarity into your mind, your head and then your neck and shoulders. As it moves through you, it carries away any tension and tightness.

- Feel the warmth of this light as it moves into your chest and down your arms and hands, and then into your abdomen, bringing with it healing and protection.

- Next, let this Divine light move into your hips and pelvis and finally down into your legs and feet.

- Let this Divine light move through you as long as you would like it to. Continue this process until you feel totally at peace and deeply relaxed.

- Know that God is always with you, caring for you and loving you always.

## Love - The Great Healer

At the deepest spiritual and emotional level, our purpose in life is to express our love and appreciation for ourselves, our family, friends, co-workers, and the entire world and all of God's creatures that we share this world with. Love has tremendous healing power and can enable us to overcome anxiety and stress better than any other emotion. When you connect with the love that lies within your heart and express it often to those around you, you will be positively transformed. It allows us to reach out beyond our own concerns and upsets and focus on loving and caring for others. There is also no other emotion that is more immensely self-nurturing and self-healing.

As a physician, I have seen the healing power of love many times. I have always been touched by the great care and acts of helpfulness that many of my women patients show to their children, spouses, other family members, and friends when they're ill. It has always heartened me to see families gather together and support a loved one who is ailing.

I have found that people tend to heal much faster and more completely when they're supported by love and caring. This is not just my own belief; many studies attest to the importance of love and positive relationships in creating health and wellness.

Conversely, I have seen feelings of anxiety, fear and other intense negative emotions literally wreak havoc on patients' physical and chemical well-being. Many patients I work with have themselves linked their poor immunity, menstrual disorders, digestive upset, high blood pressure, aching joints, and a host of other ailments to the negative and upsetting emotions they were feeling at the time. Many research studies also confirm the negative health effects that emotions like anger, depression, and loneliness cause. These studies find social isolation and lack of close relationships—the inability to connect with others in a loving way—also increases the likelihood of illness. Cultivating your love, caring and compassion are the greatest antidotes for all of these issues.

## Follow Your Heart

Follow your heart in everything you do. It is important to make all of your choices out of love, kindness, and joy. These heartfelt emotions are just as important in making decisions about your life as the logical arguments and rationalizations generated by your mind. It is the love that is centered in your heart that responds to the deepest yearnings of your soul—enabling you to create a happy and meaningful life.

The crucial role your heart plays in creating your consciousness differs from the principles of conventional Western medicine, which greatly favors your brain. However, the ancient wisdom found in our spiritual traditions deems the heart as the seat of the consciousness beyond the mind. Much fascinating medical and scientific research is now confirming this connection. There are many wonderful verses on the importance of our hearts in blessing our lives in the Bible. Here are a few of these inspiring:

1 Samuel 16:7 "Man looks at the outward appearance, but the Lord looks at the heart."

Psalm 19:8 "The precepts of the Lord are right, giving joy to the heart. The commands of the Lord are radiant, giving light to the eyes."

Psalm 51:10 "Create in me a pure heart, O God, and renew a steadfast spirit within me."

Proverbs 15:30 "A cheerful look brings joy to the heart, and good news gives health to the bones. "

Mathew 5:8 "Blessed are the pure in heart for they will see God."

Mark 12:30 "Love the Lord your God with all your heart and with all your soul and with all your mind and with all your strength….and to love your neighbor as yourself."

## *Thoughts on Love*

I want to share these heartfelt thoughts about love with you. When you do any meditations, find a quiet place where you can sit comfortably. Close your eyes, and let your arms rest easily at your side. As you take a deep breath, focus on the area of your heart (located just to the left of the center of your chest).

### At One With Life

No matter where love comes from or how it manifests, it is important for you to remember who you are. You are a beloved child of God

### Feeling Love

Focus on the people and things in your life that you love. Perhaps it is your children, your significant other or your best friend. Maybe you love your faithful dog or cat or even your favorite garden. Focus on how all of these beloved things make you feel. Enjoy the feelings of warmth and happiness that come from focusing on love.

### Accepting Love

For many women, the giving of love is easier than the accepting of love. Love can be tied to vulnerability, and, if you are struggling with anxiety and stress, what a scary place this can be. It is important to remember that love itself cannot harm you. True love is patient, generous, compassionate and kind

## Loving Visualization

I want to share a loving visualization with you. It is meant to give you a few minutes to turn inward and get back in touch with loving yourself through self-nurturance. This will help you release any negative thoughts or upsets you may have accumulated throughout the day and help you reconnect with the healing power of love.

To do this visualization, find a quiet spot where you can sit or lie comfortably. As you take a deep breath, focus on the area of your heart (located just to the left of the center of your chest).

- As you inhale and exhale slowly and deeply, close your eyes and envision your heart as a luminous, emerald green jewel glowing with love and sending out brilliant light from behind your breastbone, where your heart resides.

- As you breathe slowly, begin to fill your heart with love. Feel the area surrounding your heart soften and expand as you fill it with loving and peaceful energy.

- Then, send love and appreciation to every part of your body, even the parts that you are concerned about or feel are less than lovable. They are all parts of you and worthy of the deepest love and caring.

- Breathe love and appreciation into your head, neck, shoulders, chest and down your arms and hands.

- Send this loving and healing breath next into your abdomen, hips, legs and feet.

- Continue loving and appreciating yourself until you feel your entire body overflowing with love.

- Now, gently open your eyes and slowly begin to move around again. Enjoy the feelings of love, peace and gratitude you have created.

## Embrace Gratitude and Appreciation

As a healer, I have been very impressed by how much feelings of gratitude and appreciation have greatly reduced the level of anxiety and stress and improved the health, well-being, and quality of life for my patients over the years. These are positive qualities that I always strive to find in myself and express to everyone around me on a daily basis.

However, I did not discover any real research that had been done in this area until the some years ago. At that time, I was introduced to the innovative and groundbreaking work that was taking place at the Institute of HeartMath (IHM) in Boulder Creek, California.

Early one morning I received a call from a medical laboratory that wanted to introduce me to their facilities and services. In the course of the conversation, they told me about very exciting research they were doing with the Institute. Specifically, laboratory testing was confirming that individuals who used techniques developed by the Institute to help them alleviate their feelings of anger, stress and upset, and convert these emotions into feelings of gratitude and appreciation, were having dramatic improvements in several important chemical indicators of good health. From a medical perspective, these findings had amazing implications.

I was so intrigued by the work being done at the Institute that I called and requested their literature and research studies. After carefully reading their findings and conclusions, I was even more convinced of what I had been observing with my patients and myself—that there is a very strong, medically sound connection between positive emotions, such as gratitude, and good health.

The researchers at the IHM found that the heart plays a far more central role in stress, mental and emotional balance, and perception than previously thought. They found that the heart initiates most of the repetitious patterns within the body, and has a much more intricate communication pattern with the brain than does any other major organ.

Plus, the heart not only responds to any stimulus the brain processes— from thoughts and emotions to light and sound—it also generates many times more electrical power than the brain. The signal is so strong that the current sent out by the heart radiates throughout the body. For all these reasons, the heart is in a unique position to connect the mind, body, and spirit.

To test this theory, researchers fed two groups of rabbits a diet that was high in fat. Rabbits from the first group were held, petted, and talked to, while those in the other group were treated normally and were not shown any affection. Interestingly, they found that the rabbits that had been treated lovingly developed significantly less atherosclerosis than those rabbits that had not.

Based on this and other research, the IHM developed specific techniques to stop negative thoughts that would normally engender anxiety, fear and worry and convert them to positive feelings or emotions. By learning to generate feelings of sincere love, gratitude, and appreciation, a person's pulse, respiration, and brain wave frequencies are better able to synchronize.

In order to examine the health benefits of these techniques, the researchers then did a series of fascinating studies in which they taught these techniques to volunteers, then measured changes in various physical and chemical parameters. The results were very promising, as volunteers had more harmonious and efficient functioning of their cardiovascular, immune, and hormonal systems.

Most telling is that the people who have become adept at using these techniques have reported dramatic increases in the ability to solve problems and handle stresses such as conflicts on the job, rush hour traffic, and rebellious children.

The IHM found that appreciation can significantly increase your body's production of the steroid hormone DHEA. This is particularly exciting for women wanting to improve their hormonal health and balance. Researchers took DHEA samples from 28 volunteers, then asked them to listen to music specifically designed to promote a sense of peacefulness and emotional balance every day for one month.

At the end of the month, researchers took a second DHEA sample from the volunteers. The results were impressive. Among all volunteers, DHEA levels increased, on average, 100 percent; for some, the levels tripled and even quadrupled. This is extremely important for female hormonal balance, since DHEA is converted within your body to estrogen and testosterone.

In addition, the researchers found that feelings of care and appreciation can boost levels of an immune antibody called IgA, which is an important part of your body's defense against bacteria and viruses. And while anger is known to suppress your immune system, they discovered that even remembering a previous angry experience had a negative, long-term impact on immune function.

### Conventional Medicine Weighs In

Interestingly, the *American Journal of Cardiology* also featured a study that found that gratitude and appreciation might be positively associated with a reduction in blood pressure. However, it was several years before another mainstream medical journal would present additional support for the Institute of HeartMath's findings.

In a study from the *Journal of Social and Clinical Psychology*, researchers divided volunteers into three groups. The first group kept a daily log of five complaints, the second group wrote down a daily list of five things they were better at/did better than their peers, and the third group kept a daily log of five things they were grateful for. After three weeks, those who kept the gratitude journal reported increased energy, less health complaints, and greater feelings of overall well-being as compared to the participants in the other two groups.

This finding was corroborated in the *Journal of Personality and Social Psychology* when researchers found that many of their subjects used gratitude as a positive way to cope with acute and chronic life stressors.

## Express Your Gratitude

Journaling is a fantastic way to express your feelings of gratitude and appreciation. In her book Simple Abundance, author Sarah Ban Breathnach talks about a "gratitude journal." She recommends that you write down at least five things each day that you are thankful for, thereby forcing you to focus on what is going right in your life rather than what is going wrong. I couldn't agree with her more. Regardless of the type of journal you choose to keep, there are a few things to keep in mind:

- Select any kind of journal you want. Some women have used spiral notebooks, others a loose-leaf notebook, still others a gold-trimmed, bound book. What you choose is up to you.

- Make an appointment with yourself for fifteen minutes to half an hour each day to write.

- Choose a safe, calming location where you can write freely, without being disturbed.

- Do not censor yourself as you write - write down your emotions, good and bad. Once the thoughts and feelings are on paper, you can always throw them out if you choose to. The important thing is to get them out.

- Do not worry about punctuation or grammar.

- Finally, be free, be honest, be candid — be yourself.

Similarly, one of my favorite books is *The Art of Thank You: Crafting Notes of Gratitude* (Beyond Words Publishing, Inc.). This beautiful book suggests sending thank you notes as a way to show generosity, gratitude, and kindness to others. Why not show the same consideration to yourself? Why not start each day thanking and appreciating your body? Your family and friends?

Write these positive thank yous and appreciative thoughts as affirmations in your journal, say them out loud in the privacy of your bedroom or office, or even visualize sending loving messages to your body each day. Over time, releasing more and more of your own toxic emotions and replacing them with kind and loving thoughts to yourself will help to diminish the load on your body, mind, and spirit. Then your body will begin to be filled with the most wonderful light, radiance, and health.

### *Love and Gratitude Meditation*

This is a great meditation to do to help you reconnect with the healing power of love, forgiveness, and gratitude.

1. Find a quiet spot where you can sit or lie comfortably.

2. Close your eyes, and let your arms rest easily at your side. As you take a deep breath, focus on the area of your heart (located just to the left of the center of your chest).

3. As you slowly inhale and exhale, imagine you're filling your heart with love. Feel the area surrounding your heart soften and expand as you fill it with loving and peaceful energy.

4. Now, direct your breath into all of the parts of your body, starting with your feet and moving up through your body, finally into your head and neck.

Notice any areas where you have stored any negative or upsetting emotions such as frustration, anger, or other feelings that make certain parts of your body feel tense, tight, heavy, or devitalized.

Keep breathing love into those parts of your body until they, too, relax and soften. By the time you're done, you should feel much more quiet and peaceful.

5. Now visualize your love radiating out from you and touching everyone you love and care about. If you choose to, you can send your love and the spirit of healing to your community, to our country, and even the entire earth.

6. Now gently open your eyes and slowly begin to move around again. Enjoy the feelings of love, peace, and gratitude you have created.

## Practice Forgiveness

Practicing forgiveness of others is essential to transforming anxiety and stress into a greater sense of peace, calm and relaxation. In my practice, I've seen conditions as diverse as heart disease, high blood pressure, arthritis, inflammation, allergies, and immune disorders aggravated by frequent and constant feelings of resentment and anger. I've also seen unresolved and unexpressed anger contribute to menstrual problems, excessive weight gain and a host of other physical ailments.

In fact, several studies have also linked anger to neck and backaches, muscle tension, elevated homocysteine levels, and increased progression of coronary atherosclerosis. If you too suffer from unresolved anger and illnesses that can result from keeping it bottled up inside, then take heart. It is possible for you to release the offensive feelings and move forward with your life.

## Erin's Story

I was recently chatting with my friend Erin who shared with me that anger was the one emotion she was always afraid to express. Several decades ago, Erin's mother and aunt had a major disagreement. They didn't speak to one another for years, and never had the opportunity to reconcile before the aunt's death.

Over time, Erin began to equate expressing anger or upset with a loss of love or friendship. As a result, she has held in any resentment or frustration she has felt toward those close to her rather than express her feelings to her family or friends. The idea of expressing her angry and upsetting feelings and losing love as a result made her feel constantly anxious and fearful.

The irony is that the only one affected was Erin. The people she was angry with went about their daily lives completely unaffected and unaware of Erin's anxiety and stress over her unexpressed upset In addition, her anxiety caused worsening hot flashes, chronic headaches, digestive upset and emotional paralysis. As Erin finally began to forgive the people she had so much upset with, let go of her anger and start to express her emotions, her feelings of anxiety began to diminish and her physical symptoms began to ease up.

Strange as it may sound, many women are hesitant to let go of their anger and resentment. Not only is it hard for many of us to forgive others, but it is difficult to forgive ourselves for our own personal faults and weaknesses. Frequently, anger becomes a comfortable, familiar barrier between you and disappointment or upset. But trust me when I tell you that the only way for good, positive changes to come into your life is for you to take action now to forgive the person who wronged you, forgive yourself, and move on.

Once you empower yourself to take charge of and responsibility for your emotional responses, the rewards will come pouring in. You may reconcile and heal relationships that have been tainted by resentment, anger, and pain. Marriages, families, and friendships that have been strained for years may improve. You could lose unwanted weight or lessen the frequency of debilitating headaches. But most importantly, your quality of life will drastically improve, providing you with greater peace, contentment, and optimism in your life and in your relationships.

If you have a problem dealing with or letting go of resentment, anger, and pain—and forgiving yourself and those you perceive as having hurt you—here are a few suggestions to help you start turning that pattern around quickly and effectively:

1. When you feel upset, learn to express your feelings quickly, in a way that allows you to find positive solutions to your grievances. This will help you to resolve situations that you may have felt stuck in for years, and regain more hope and joy in your life with all of your relationships. Then learn to focus on your appreciation of others, rather than on what angers or upsets you.

2. The most powerful antidotes to anger are the words "I forgive you," "I appreciate you," and "thank you." Learn to say and feel these words often to the people and situations in your life.

3. Look at the positive aspects of your life rather than feeling angry and resentful for what you feel you don't have or what you lack. This will also help you to heal long-standing hurts.

4. If your relationships with certain people or situations turn out to be unworkable and only trigger anger and upset rather than happiness or pleasure, consider gently and lovingly letting them go from your life rather than staying stuck in constant anger or upset.

### Change the Anger to Appreciation

The following affirmations take about one minute to do, but can have lifelong benefits. Keep them nearby and repeat them any time you feel anger and resentment building up inside of you.

1. I enjoy focusing on and giving thanks for all of the many positive people and situations in my life.

2. When people or situations cause me to feel upset, I look for positive ways to deal with my grievances so that I feel pleased with the outcome.

3. I seek to deal with the upsets and challenges in my life with a sense of calm and peacefulness.

4. I communicate my feelings of anger and upset when necessary in a kind and thoughtful way that will do no harm to myself or others.

5. I let go of resentment and don't allow it to accumulate inside of me.

6. I enjoy finding new ways to make my life even more positive and joyful.

7. I forgive all of those people who have caused me to feel upset and angry in the past.

8. I forgive myself.

## *A Blessing for Appreciation*

Each day, it is very beneficial to take your focus off of anxiety, fear and worry and instead give appreciation to those you love and cherish. I recommend sharing the following words of gratitude:

- Thank you for being there for me.

- Thank you for caring.

- Thank you for listening to me during my times of need.

- Thank you for your kind touch.

- Thank you for your love.

## Live for Laughter

I absolutely love to laugh and always enjoy finding the fun and lightness in every situation that I can in my life. I think it's one of the most powerful and effective healing tools there are. There is no doubt that positive emotions like laughter and joy have tremendous health benefits — plus, they make your life more wondrous and enjoyable.

I have found that boosting your daily laughter is a great way to release anxiety and relax the tensions we are holding. That's why I developed the stress-to-laughter index. It comes from observing the stories my patients have shared with me over the years, as well as examining my own life and those of my friends and family. And what I've seen is that this index can really help you judge how effectively you are providing stress relief for yourself.

If you have too much anxiety, fear, worry, heaviness, seriousness or concerns and not enough fun and laughter in your life, it's time to flip the scales in the other direction. I've seen thousands of cases of patients getting flare-ups of illnesses, such as colds, flus, immune breakdowns, worsening of menopause symptoms, menstrual cramps, PMS, and painful arthritic episodes immediately following periods of too much stress and heaviness in their lives.

Often, just by flipping into a state of laughter and fun, you can help to bring yourself back into a state of optimal health. Anxiety and stress are diminished, your immune system functions better, your hormones are more likely to be in balance, and pain is reduced when you laugh and have fun, thanks to a whole cascade of positive chemicals within your body that are released during times of joy and fun.

To this point, I can distinctly remember a time I was working too much and was feeling a lot of anxiety and pressure over meeting deadlines. I noticed that it began to have negative effects on my body. I was waking up in the morning feeling stiff, my neck was tense, and my muscles were tight. I also noticed that I wasn't digesting my food quite as well. In short, I was pushing myself to a place of too much stress. I quickly realized that it was time for me to give myself a big dose of laughter, fun, and pleasure to bring myself into healthy balance.

I decided to take a break from my busy routine and take my daughter to the local toy store and have some fun. We bought paint, drawing materials, puzzles and other toys. When we came home, we laid our treasures out on the dining room table, then spent the entire evening playing with our paints, toys and games. It was definitely the right antidote for me and helped me release my anxiety and stress over my work deadlines and get back into balance.

I noticed that with all of the joy and laughter, my muscles started to loosen up and feel better. The next morning, I woke up and felt much more refreshed, light, and energetic. I even found that I was digesting my food normally again. In short, laughter truly is the best medicine.

## Mainstream Medicine Has a Sense of Humor

The healing power of laughter has been the subject of many studies. According to an article published in *Family Practice News*, children laugh, on average, about 400 times a day, while adults only laugh about 15 times a day. This is a sad state of affairs, because when laughter is your automatic response to stress, trying times are less likely to feel anxious and fearful.

Dr. Norman Cousins introduced this concept to medicine after he was diagnosed with a severe health condition called ankylosing spondylitis. He was determined to find a treatment for his disabling condition, and essentially cured himself by listening to recordings of laughter, watching lots of funny movies, and taking large doses of vitamin C.

More recently, research studies have provided scientific confirmation of this phenomenon. Laughter has been shown to lower the stress hormone cortisol, as well as blood pressure and heart rate, and to increase mood-elevating beta-endorphins—natural, feel-good chemicals produced by your body that are 200 times more potent than morphine.

And when it comes to smiles, it turns out they really are contagious. Researchers at the University of California at San Francisco determined that there are 19 different kinds of smiles, all of which are extremely contagious! In addition, Russian research has found that frequent smiling helps people heal from a host of degenerative diseases.

Whatever your sense of humor calls for, indulge it. Go on a laughter odyssey and discover what tickles your funny bone. Whether you like to watch silly movies, read funny books, tell or listen to jokes, visit a comedy club, play games, or go to the toy store, I strongly recommend that you enjoy a little levity as often as possible. And always try to see the humor in the little frustrations and minor disasters that occur every day. It can greatly improve the quality of your life, and just might even save it!

## Hold on to Happiness

Your state of health is very closely tied to how truly happy you are. A study on this important subject, published in the *Proceedings of the National Academy of Sciences*, found that people who consider themselves happy are more likely to be healthy and resistant to disease. They also have lower levels of the stress hormone cortisol and a reduced risk of heart disease. This study joins an ever-growing body of research that proves the importance of creating a life in which positive feelings of love, happiness, joy, and optimism predominate over negativity.

There is one particular study I love. Researchers studied the longevity of a group of 178 Catholic nuns from a convent in Milwaukee. The nuns lived together and taught in the same school. They had the same daily routine, ate the same food, didn't smoke or drink alcohol, had the same financial situation, and had identical medical care.

The researchers then looked at the writings each nun did prior to taking her vows. A separate team of psychologists then assessed the positive and negative comments made in the writings, and divided the sisters into different classifications based on the degree of joy and satisfaction in their letters.

The researchers then took these classifications and matched them against the life spans of each of the nuns. They found that 90 percent of those nuns who fell into the "most happy" category were still alive at 85 years old. Conversely, only 34 percent of those who were categorized as "least happy" lived to be 85.

Other studies have shown comparable results. A two-year study of 2,000 people over the age of 65 found that the mortality rate of those people who expressed the most negative emotions was twice as high as those who expressed positive emotions. Similarly, a study from Finland discovered that of the 96,000 widowed people surveyed, the surviving spouse's risk of dying doubled in the week following their spouse's death.

## *Attributes of Happy People*

In the following list, I share many attributes of happy people. If you don't recognize yourself in at least three or four, aim to practice these principles so you can become "One of the Happiest People You Know."

1. Appreciate the many blessings that you already have in your life. When you focus on the positives in your life, it will draw even more to you!

2. Find something to love, appreciate and admire about everyone—and everything—in your life. Have a genuine sense of self-worth and always look for the good in others.

3. Know that you can choose to let go of feelings of worry and fear and replace them with feelings of positivity, optimism, confidence and "can do" about working through any of your life's challenges.

4. View life through the eyes of awe and wonder like a small child. Know beyond a shadow of a doubt that all things are truly possible.

5. Briefly acknowledge what you don't want, and then identify what you prefer instead. Use your innate creativity to chart a path to find ways to manifest these positive preferences.

6. Totally let go things that no longer serve you. Feelings and emotions like fear, worry, resentment, anger, judgment, criticism, guilt, shame and blame have no place in your life. When you release and let go of these emotional burdens, you can replace them with the wonderful qualities of love, joy, acceptance, peace, caring, compassion and happiness.

7. Cultivate patience. Rather than judging people for what they haven't accomplished, support them in the positive attributes that they have now.

8. Love others unconditionally, even when others are less than loving toward you. Over time, this will create positive change within the relationship. I have seen this happen very often when seemingly "hopeless" relationships transform into kind, loving and nurturing friendships and family relationships.

## Accentuate the Positive

I'm sure you've heard the expression "do unto others as you would have them do unto you." I think this is a wonderful credo to live by. Unfortunately, in my experience, many women seem to have an easier time with "unto others" than with "unto yourself."

So often I hear women say things about themselves, their bodies, and even their talents, which seem to be self-denigrating. We are constantly criticizing ourselves for not being good enough, smart enough, beautiful enough, or thin enough. My women friends are always jokingly offering to give each other transplants of their most disliked body parts—usually the breasts, behinds, and stomachs. This can create a great deal of anxiety and stress and undermine your sense of confidence about yourself if you practice this mindset.

It makes me wonder why this trait is so common among women, and what, if anything, we can do to treat ourselves in a more accepting, caring, and nurturing way. Much of this stems from childhood, when women are often programmed for self-criticism by hearing their own mothers' subtle (or not so subtle) messages of feeling somehow unworthy in their own lives—no matter how accomplished we or our mothers actually are. My own mother, who was a beautiful and accomplished woman and also a medical doctor, did this when I was growing up. This is how deeply negative programming can reach!

Add to this society's impossible standards regarding how a woman should look-- rail-thin, with flawless skin and perfectly coiffed hair—and it should come as no surprise that most women are in a constant self-dialogue of criticism and scorn.

## *Stop the Negative Self-Talk*

When this type of negative self-talk becomes the norm rather than the exception, it can become downright abusive. I'm not referring to physical abuse, but a tendency for a woman to turn emotional violence on herself. Before you wave this off as something that doesn't apply to you, ask yourself these questions:

1. Do you set impossibly high standards for yourself?

2. Do you have higher expectations of yourself than of others?

3. Do you see a friend as "pleasantly plump" but yourself as obese?

4. Do you fixate on a particular aspect of your appearance that most people probably don't even notice?

5. Do you find that if a friend or loved one makes a mistake, or does something hurtful or unwise, you have compassion for her, but if you do something similar, you think of yourself as "stupid" "a loser" or a "failure"?

If you can take an objective look in the mirror and admit that you are harder on yourself than you are on anybody else in your life, then you are at an emotional fork in the road. And there's more at stake than your self-esteem. In fact, the path you choose may determine your level of anxiety and stress and even your physical health.

Research has repeatedly linked our level of self-esteem to emotional and physical well-being. According to a study published in the *Journal of Aging and Health*, positive psychological states and self-image were actually protective against health problems in older adults. Similarly, research from the *Journal of the American Medical Association* found that negative emotions, such as self-criticism, can cause a reduction in blood flow to the heart. And, a study in the *British Journal of Psychiatry* found a higher risk of depression in women with a negative self-image.

## Start Loving Yourself

For optimal emotional and physical health, it's important that you send positive messages to your body that reinforce your sense of self-worth and self-love. Try to put to rest any emotional issues you have that are chronic and self-destructive in nature, such as self-criticism and setting yourself up for a lifetime of failures by setting standards that no woman could possibly achieve.

The trouble is most women have tried to live up to unrealistic expectations for so long that the concept of self-deprecation has become deeply ingrained in their minds. As a result, even when you intellectually understand that you need to stop being so hard on yourself, in many cases you find that you simply can't stop. The habit of putting yourself down is so embedded in your mind that the self-destructive thought processes and behaviors have become an involuntary reflex.

My colleague Stacey is a good example. Stacey is a highly accomplished and successful woman. She has an Ivy League doctoral degree, seven published books, hundreds of magazine and scholarly journal articles to her credit, and has been happily married for more than 30 years. She also has a negative and sad secret: She believes she's unworthy and not good enough. She thinks she's the only one who knows, and she works hard to keep it that way. If someone asks her a question, she diligently researches the answer rather than admitting she doesn't know. If she makes a mistake, everything she's ever done right pales in comparison. If someone criticizes her, she can't get it out of her mind.

Contrast Stacey with the mother of one of my college friends. When you were around Rachel, she made you think she was absolutely the most beautiful woman in the world. However, she wasn't particularly attractive in a conventional sense. In fact, some people might have considered her dowdy and plain.

A wise and perceptive woman who was a close friend of the family told me a bit about Rachel's background. She grew up poor, with parents who had very little education. Yet she was an extremely accomplished woman in both her professional and personal life. She had several advanced academic degrees, a high-powered career, and a husband, family, and friends who adored her. Most fascinating to me, however, was the sheer joy she took in herself and everyone around her. It was infectious, and she made us all feel good when we were in her presence.

What's her secret? According to the family friend, despite their own lack of wealth and accomplishment, Rachel's parents had told her from day one how beautiful, capable, and intelligent she was, and that she could achieve anything she wanted. It was a wonderful, positive programming that imprinted Rachel in the deepest way. The good news is that you can create this positive programming, too, no matter what your age or what you perceive are the level of accomplishments in your own life!!

As these two stories show, the key to loving yourself is to reprogram your mind with a new belief system. To do this, you need to redefine your circle of loved ones to include one very special, important, and hard working person—YOU!

## Self-Loving Affirmations

I want to share with you a few positive affirmations that reinforce your self-love and self-worth. I use them for loving and honoring myself, too. I encourage you to use them to enhance your feelings of self-love and value.

To begin, place your hands in prayer position over your heart. Close your eyes and fill you mind with the most beautiful, peaceful image you can.

Repeat the affirmations five times each. When you feel emotion welling up in your eyes, you'll know that the message got in.

1. I honor and love myself.

2. I am enough.

3. I treat myself with kindness, gentleness, and nurturing.

4. I am worthy.

5. The Divine light of God protects and nurtures me in every way.

6. Every day, I fill myself with feelings of love for God, my friends and family, and all people and creatures on Earth.

7. Kindness and compassion for myself softens and illuminates my heart, casting a warm glow on the world around me.

8. I recognize the light of God in myself, those close to me, and in everyone I encounter on my life journey.

9. I rely on my inner reserves of courage and self-confidence to help make the right choices and decisions.

10. My heart is filled with appreciation and gratitude for all of the blessings that have been bestowed upon me.

## The Gift of Giving

Practicing giving to others with a spirit of generosity is a quality that can uplift your spirit and improve your mood. Abundance can manifest many ways, not just financially. You can also feel abundant in your joy, your love and your personal relationships to such an extent that you can pass the overflow on to others.

An act of generosity implies having trust that there is more than enough to go around, as well as confidence in your own inner emotional abundance. It is a great antidote to anxiety and stress because it takes our mind off of our own fears and worries and, instead, focuses our attention in a loving way on the needs of others.

Generosity can be physical in which we share our physical belongings with other in need, whether that be money, food, clothing or the gift of our time. It can also be emotional generosity when we make others feel good and worthy, despite feelings that we may sometimes have to the contrary.

I want to share a story of generosity with you that one of my friends and colleagues, David, shared with me. "One night when leaving the hospital with a small group of friends, a woman asked for help in jumping her car battery. After 30 minutes of unsuccessful attempts, I had to leave to attend a prior engagement.

Thankfully, several friends were able to stay on with her. After concluding that her battery was dead, they gave her a ride to her sister's house and then picked up a new car battery with her and drove her back to the hospital where her car was parked. They installed the car battery for her and made sure she was able to get back safely on the road.

After spending several hours helping her, she was completely amazed and touched that strangers would assist her to this extent, without asking for anything in return, no strings attached or preaching. Just "We're glad you are safe and back on the road." I was very touched by their heartfelt generosity when David told me this story

My friend, Jane, is a great example of transforming a negative feeling or reaction into a positive feeling of acceptance for another person and behaving with a spirit of kindness and generosity. Recently, Jane stopped at a local restaurant on her way home from work to pick up dinner for her family. She was feeling guilty about feeding them fast food for the third time that week, but she was running late, her husband was due at a meeting in an hour, and she'd had a particularly hard day.

When she arrived at the counter, the waitress who was supposed to be taking her order was chatting on her cell phone. Jane could tell that the woman had seen her out of the corner of her eye, but she just kept on talking. Finally, after what seemed like an eternity later, she hung up, turned to Jane and said, "What can I get you?" At this point, Jane was so frustrated and angry that she wanted to verbally assault the woman, but she realized that she had a window of opportunity to make a choice: She could fire off a sarcastic comment to mirror her self-righteous anger but she knew that it would unleash a flood of stress hormones into her system.

She realized that her blood pressure was already too high, her stomach was in a knot, and she didn't need her headache to get worse. She also knew that she'd feel bad about losing her temper later on. She decided to reframe her feelings into positive acceptance of the woman in front of her so she took a deep breath, gave her a big, genuine smile and placed her order. Just then her waitress apologized and told Jane that she was on the phone with her family because her mother was ill. Jane expressed her concern for the woman's mother and ended up giving her a big hug. By the time she left with her food, she was feeling much better about herself and the world, in general.

Jane's response ended up being generous to both herself and the woman taking the order. It was generous to be kind and understanding and not to strike out verbally, as she initially felt like doing. It was generous to spare herself the consequences of a flood of stress hormones and remorse. And it was generous to her family not to bring home dinner with a side order of anger and resentment energetically contaminating the food. Instead, she made a positive offering of love.

## The Research Tells the Story

Harvard researchers have studied the effects of altruism by taking before-and-after measurements of immune system markers in the saliva of volunteers who watched three films: the first on gardening, the second about war, and the third about Mother Teresa. There was no change in immune markers before or after the first two films, but after the third one, a marker for improved immune function rose dramatically. In other words, just watching someone else be generous is good for your health.

In another landmark study, a researcher from the University of Michigan followed 2,700 people for more than a decade to determine how their social relationships affected their health. He found that more than any other activity, doing volunteer work improved health and increased life expectancy.

Psychologists Allan Luks and Howard Andrews collected surveys from more than 3,000 student volunteers and found that their "helper's high" was followed by a second stage they called the "healthy-helper syndrome." They defined this stage as "a longer-lasting sense of calm and heightened emotional well-being... that is a powerful antidote to anxiety and stress, a key to happiness and optimism, and a way to combat feelings of helplessness and depression."

## You Get What You Give

Generosity has a ripple effect—it's contagious. When you give to someone else, they're more likely to give to others. Small acts of generosity, those practiced during your day-to-day life, have a more far-reaching impact than you could ever imagine. When you stop to assist a lone person whose car has broken down and is in obvious distress or help an elderly and unsteady person cross the street, the feel-good endorphins you just created for yourself and someone else will be passed on, possibly to hundreds or even thousands of others. If you could actually follow the ripple effects of your acts of generosity, you would see that they go on forever. In essence, you've just thrown your coin into the cosmic river of life!

# 9

## Relaxation Techniques for Relief of Anxiety and Stress

Practicing relaxation exercises is a very effective way to help deal with the day-to-day stresses that can often increase your feelings of anxiety and nervous tension. If you have a healthy emotional balance, you can more easily handle minor everyday pressures. These daily stresses, however, can feel overwhelming if your anxiety responses are easily triggered. Such stress can include riding in an elevator, being in crowds, going to the dentist, or any situation, place, or person that sparks a woman's emotional charge. Often these charged issues evoke anxiety, fear, or upset feelings.

Moreover, significant lifestyle changes—death of a loved one, divorce, job loss, financial problems, major changes in personal relationships—can be almost impossible to handle if you are already feeling anxious and tense. Being unable to cope with stress effectively can also damage your self-esteem and self-confidence. When you suffer from frequent anxiety episodes, you may feel a decreasing sense of self-worth as your ability to handle your usual range of activities diminishes. These are often complaints that I hear from my patients. Perhaps these are issues for you, too. Our life stresses don't necessarily change, so how well you cope with them can really make a positive difference.

In this chapter, I will be sharing with you many wonderful and very effective stress relieving and relaxation exercises to help retrain your mind, emotions and stress response towards more balance, peace and equanimity when facing life's challenges.

Let's look now at how stress affects your body.

## How Stress Affects the Body

Your emotional and physical reactions to stress are partly determined by the sensitivity of your sympathetic nervous system. This system produces the fight-or-flight reaction in response to stress and excitement, speeding up and heightening the pulse rate, respiration, muscle tension, glandular function, and circulation of the blood.

If you have recurrent anxiety symptoms, either major or minor lifestyle and emotional upsets may cause an overreaction of your sympathetic system. If you have an especially stressful life, your sympathetic nervous system may always be poised to react to a crisis, putting you in a state of constant tension. In this mode, you tend to react to small stresses the same way you would react to real emergencies. The energy that accumulates in the body to meet this "emergency" must be discharged in order to bring your body back into balance.

Repeated episodes of the fight-or-flight reaction deplete your energy reserves and, if they continue, cause a downward spiral that can lead to emotional burnout and eventually complete exhaustion. You can break this spiral only by learning to manage stress in a way that protects and even increases your energy level.

## Techniques for Relaxation

Many patients have asked me about techniques for coping more effectively with stress. Although I send some women for counseling or psychotherapy when symptoms are severe, most of my patients are looking for practical ways to manage stress on their own. They want effective techniques for handling their stress response as it arises and to prevent it from recurring.

Happily, I have found that practicing the types of stress reduction techniques that I share with you in this chapter can pay great dividends, especially when practiced on a regular basis

I have included relaxation and stress reduction exercises in many of my patient programs. The feedback has been very positive. Many of my patients have reported an increased sense of well-being from these relaxation exercises and meditations. They have also noted an improvement in their physical health and energy levels.

This chapter includes fourteen stress-reduction exercises for you to work with and enjoy. They will take you through a series of specific steps to help alleviate your symptoms. The exercises will teach you the following helpful techniques: focusing and meditation, grounding techniques (how to feel more centered), exercises that help you to relax and release muscle tension, erasure techniques (how to erase old emotions), healing the inner child, visualizations, and affirmations.

These techniques will help you cope with stress more efficiently. They will make your thoughts more positive and optimistic as well as engender feelings of peace and calm. These exercises will help you learn to relax while you build self-esteem and self-confidence.

You may want to begin by trying them all or you can do the ones that appeal to you the most. I recommend that you practice the ones that produce the most anxiety relieving benefits on a regular basis.

## Quieting the Mind and Body

Women with recurring symptoms of anxiety and nervous tension are usually barraged by a constant stream of negative "self-talk." Throughout the day your conscious mind may be inundated with thoughts, feelings, and fantasies that trigger feelings of upset. Many of these thoughts replay unresolved issues of health, finances, or personal and work relationships. This relentless mental replay of unresolved issues can reinforce the anxiety symptoms and be exhausting. It is important to know how to shut off the constant inner dialogue and quiet your mind.

The first two meditation exercises require you to sit quietly and engage in a simple repetitive activity. By emptying your mind, you give your brain and mind a rest. Meditation allows you to create a state of deep relaxation, which is very healing to the entire body. Metabolism slows, as do physiological functions such as heart rate and blood pressure. Muscle tension decreases. Brain wave patterns shift from the fast beta waves that occur during a normal active day to the slower alpha waves, which appear just before falling asleep or in times of deep relaxation. If you practice these exercises regularly, they can help relieve anxiety by resting your mind and turning off upsetting thoughts.

The third meditation will help you release tension and relax. If you want to enjoy deep restful sleep, this peaceful meditation will help you relax and unwind. I've seen it create great benefits for both adults and children, alike. It is a very simple, yet effective, exercise.

### Exercise 1: Focusing

Select a small personal object that you like a great deal. It might be a jeweled pin or a simple flower from your garden. Focus all your attention on this object as you inhale and exhale slowly and deeply for one to two minutes.

While you are doing this exercise, try not to let any other thoughts or feelings enter your mind. If they do, just return your attention to the object.

At the end of this exercise you will probably feel more peaceful and calmer. Any tension or nervousness that you were feeling upon starting the exercise should be diminished.

## Exercise 2: Meditation on Peace

- Sit or lie in a comfortable position.

- Close your eyes and breathe deeply. Let your breathing be slow and relaxed.

- Focus all your attention on your breathing. Notice the movement of your chest and abdomen in and out.

- Block out all other thoughts, feelings, and sensations. If you feel your attention wandering, bring it back to your breathing.

- As you inhale, say the word "peace" to yourself, and as you exhale, say the word "calm." Draw out the pronunciation of the word so that it lasts for the entire breath. The word "peace" sounds like p-e-e-a-a-a-c-c-c-e-e. The word "calm" sounds like: c-a-a-a-l-l-l-l-m-m-m. Repeating these words as you breathe will help you to concentrate.

- Continue this exercise until you feel very relaxed.

## Exercise 3: Meditation for Sleep and Relaxation

To begin the meditation, breathe in and out, slowly and deeply. Let the cares of the day fall away.

Now visualize being in your favorite peaceful place, whether it is a garden, meadow, seashore or favorite getaway. Look around you and enjoy the sense of calm and relaxation that you get from being in this beautiful place. You can stay in this place of peace as long as you want.

As you continue to breathe in and out slowly and deeply, let yourself gently fall into a peaceful sleep.

## Grounding Technique

When women are feeling anxious and tense, they often lose a sense of being grounded, literally rooted to the earth. Some women report a sensation of numbness in their legs and feet. They may say that they feel as if they have no legs at all. Perhaps you have experienced these sensations, too, during times of stress.

When you become physically ungrounded by symptoms of emotional distress, it is also difficult to function mentally. You can have a hard time focusing and concentrating. There is a pervasive sense of "things falling apart." You may even have difficulty working through your projects for the day in an organized manner. When anxiety episodes occur, it often takes a concentrated effort just to get through the day, accomplishing such basic daily tasks as cooking, house cleaning, taking care of children, or getting to work or school.

This next exercise will help you to ground and focus both physically and mentally. Practicing this exercise will allow you to organize your energies and proceed more effectively with your daily routine during times when you feel more anxious and scattered. You should feel much more stable and focused by the end of this exercise.

## Exercise 4: Grounding

Sit upright in a chair. Be sure you are in a comfortable position. Keep your feet slightly apart. Breathe in and out through your nose.

- Inhale deeply. As you breathe in, allow your stomach to relax so that the air flows into your abdomen. Let your stomach balloon out as you breathe in. Visualize the lowest parts of your lungs filling up with air. Hold your inhalation.

- Visualize a golden cord with a golden ball at the end of it running from the base of your spine. Let this golden cord gently and slowly move downwards through the earth, grounding you. You can let it move down as far as you would like, even all the way to the center of the earth.

- Follow the cord and its golden ball in your mind all the way down and see it fasten securely to the earth's center. You can run two golden cords from the bottoms of your feet down to the center of the earth, also, if you would like.

- As you exhale, become aware of your hips, thighs, calves, ankles, and feet. Feel their strength and solidity.

- Repeat this exercise several times until you feel fully present and grounded.

## Releasing Muscle Tension

The next three exercises will help you get in touch with your areas of muscle tension and then help you learn to release this tension. This is an important sequence for women with emotional symptoms of anxiety and nervous tension since habitual emotional patterns cause certain muscle groups to tense and tighten.

For example, if you have difficulty in expressing feelings, your neck muscles may be chronically tense. If you are dealing with a lot of fear and worry or repressed anger, you may have episodes of chest pain and tight chest muscles during times when you are feeling upset and are having difficulty expressing it or even handling the situation that is causing these symptoms.

When blocked feelings and emotions cause your muscles to tighten and contract, this limits the movement and flow of energy in the body. Tight muscles have decreased blood circulation and oxygenation and accumulate an excess of waste products, such as carbon dioxide and lactic acid. As a result, muscle tension can be a significant cause of the fatigue that often accompanies chronic stress. The following exercises will help release tension and the blocked emotions held in tight muscles.

## Exercise 5: Discovering Muscle Tension

- Lie on your back in a comfortable position. Allow your arms to rest at your sides, palms down, on the surface next to you.

- Raise just the right hand and arm and hold it elevated for 15 seconds.

- Notice if your forearm feels tight and tense or if the muscles are soft and pliable.

- Let your hand and arm drop down and relax. The arm muscles will relax too.

- As you lie still, notice any other parts of your body that feel tense, muscles that feel tight and sore. You may notice a constant dull aching in certain muscles.


## Exercise 6: Progressive Muscle Relaxation

- Lie on your back in a comfortable position. Allow your arms to rest at your sides, palms down, on the surface next to you.

- Inhale and exhale slowly and deeply.

- Clench your hands into fists and hold them for a few seconds.

- Then let your hands relax. On relaxing, see a golden light flowing into the entire body, making all your muscles soft and pliable.

- Now, tense and relax the following parts of your body in this order: face, shoulders, back, stomach, pelvis, legs, feet, and toes. Hold each part tensed for a few seconds and then relax your body for 15 seconds before going on to the next part.

- Finish the exercise by shaking your hands and imagining the remaining tension flowing out of your fingertips.

## *Exercise 7: Release of Muscle Tension and Anxiety*

- Lie in a comfortable position. Allow your arms to rest at your sides, palms down. Inhale and exhale slowly and deeply with your eyes closed.

- Become aware of your feet, ankles, and legs. Notice if these parts of your body have any muscle tension or tightness. If so, how does the tense part of your body feel? Is it viselike, knotted, cold or numb? Do you notice any feelings, such as hurt, upset, fear or anger coming up or even just a feeling of tension as you focus on that part of your body? Breathe into that part of your body until you feel it relax. Release any feelings or emotions with your breathing, continuing until they begin to decrease in intensity and fade.

- Next, move your awareness to your hips, pelvis, and lower back. Notice any tension or anxious feelings located in that part of your body. Breathe into your hips and pelvis until you feel them relax. Release any negative emotions as you breathe in and out. You should begin to feel more peace and calm as you continue to breathe deeply and slowly, in and out.

- Focus on your abdomen and chest. Notice any tense or upset feelings located in this area and let them drop away as you breathe in and out. Continue to release any upsetting feelings located in your abdomen or chest.

- Finally, focus on your head, neck, arms, and hands. Note any tension in this area and release it. With your breathing, release any negative feelings blocked in this area until you can't feel them anymore. Let them be replaced by feelings of peace, calm and relaxation.

- When you have finished releasing tension throughout the body, continue deep breathing and relaxing for another minute or two. At the end of this exercise, you should feel lighter and more energized.

## Erasing Stress and Tension

Often the situations and beliefs that make us feel anxious, fearful and tense feel large and insurmountable. We tend to form pictures in our mind that empower stress. In these images, we look tiny and helpless, while the stressors look huge and unsolvable.

You can change these mental images and cut stressors down to size. The next two exercises will help you to gain mastery over stress by learning to shrink it or even erase it with your mind. This places stress in a much more manageable and realistic perspective and allows you to focus on creative solutions to your issues and challenges. These two exercises will help engender a sense of power and mastery, thereby reducing anxiety and restoring a sense of calm.

### Exercise 8: Shrinking Stress

- Sit or lie in a comfortable position. Breathe slowly and deeply. Visualize a situation, person, or even a belief that makes you feel anxious and tense.

- As you do this, you might see a person's face, a place you're afraid to go, or simply a dark cloud. Where do you see this stressful picture? Is it above you, to one side, or in front of you? How does it look? Is it big or little, dark or light? Does it have certain colors?

- Now slowly begin to shrink the stressful picture. Continue to see the stressful picture shrinking until it is so small that it can literally be held in the palm of your hand. Hold your hand out in front of you, and place the picture in the palm of your hand.

- Now the stressful picture is so small it can fit on your finger. Watch it shrink from there until it finally turns into a little dot and disappears.

- Often this exercise causes feelings of amusement, as well as relaxation, as the feared stressor shrinks, gets less intimidating, and finally disappears.

*Exercise 9: Erasing Stress*

- Sit or lie in a comfortable position. Breathe slowly and deeply.

- Visualize a situation, a person, or even a belief (such as, "I'm afraid to go to the shopping mall" or "I'm scared to mix with other people at parties") that causes you to feel anxious and fearful.

- As you do this you might see a specific person, an actual place, or simply shapes and colors. Where do you see this stressful picture? Is it below you, to the side, in front of you? How does it look? Is it big or little, dark or light, or does it have a specific color?

- Imagine that a large eraser, like the kind used to erase chalk marks, has just floated into your hand. Actually feel and see the eraser in your hand. Take the eraser and begin to rub it over the area where the stressful picture is located. As the eraser rubs out the stressful picture it fades, shrinks, and finally disappears. When you can no longer see the stressful picture, simply continue to focus on your deep breathing for another minute, inhaling and exhaling slowly and deeply.

- Then, see yourself handling the situation or person who formerly caused you distress with self-confidence and mastery. Know that you are empowered and capable of handling any situation that you choose and that you can create positive solutions to every perceived issue or challenge.

- Let feelings of peace and calm fill your mind as you continue to breathe slowly and deeply.

## Healing the Inner Child

Many of our anxieties and fears come from our inner child rather than our adult self. Sometimes it is difficult to realize that the emotional upsets can cause so much suffering are actually feelings left over or originate from childhood fears, traumas, and experiences. When unhealed, they remain with us into adulthood, causing emotional distress over issues that competent "grown-up" people feel they should be able to handle.

For example, fear of the dark, fear of being unlovable, and fear of rejection often originate in early dysfunctional or unhappy experiences with our parents, siblings or other relationships. They can also arise from difficult life circumstances such as family poverty or lack that we experienced when we were young.

While these deep, unresolved emotional issues may sometimes require counseling, particularly if they are causing anxiety and stress episodes, there is much that we can do for ourselves to heal childhood wounds. The next exercise helps you to get in touch with your own inner child and facilitates the healing process.

## Exercise 10: Healing the Inner Child

- Sit or lie in a comfortable position. Breathe slowly and deeply. Begin to get in touch with where your inner child resides. Is she located in your abdomen, in your chest, or by your side? (This may actually be the part of your body where you feel the most fear and anxiety) How old is she? Can you see what clothes she is wearing? What are her emotions? Is she upset, anxious, sad, or angry? Is she withdrawn and quiet?

- Now visualize holding her in your arms or putting her on your lap. See yourself cuddling her and treating her with love and tenderness. Maybe she would like a toy animal or a doll that you can give to her. If she is sad or upset, let her know how special and precious she is to you and how much you love her. Continue to hold her and cuddle or rock her in your arms until you feel her becoming more peaceful and calm.

- Then begin to fill your inner child with a peaceful, healing, golden light. Let this beautiful, loving light fills every cell in her body. Watch her body relax.

- As you leave your inner child feeling peaceful, return your focus to your breathing. Spend a minute inhaling and exhaling deeply and slowly. If you like working with your inner child, return to visit her often!

## Visualization

The next four exercises use visualization as a therapeutic method to beneficially affect the physical and mental processes of the body. The first two focus on using color. Color therapy has a long history of being used to promote healing. In many fascinating studies, scientists have exposed subjects to specific colors, either directly through exposure to light therapy, or through changing the color of their environment.

Research done throughout the world has shown that color therapy can have a profoundly positive effect on health, well-being and even affect your mood. It can stimulate the endocrine glands, the immune system, nervous system and help to balance your emotions and mood. Visualizing color in a specific part of the body can also have a powerful therapeutic effect, too, and can be a good stress management technique for relief of anxiety and nervous tension.

The first exercise uses the color blue, which provides a calming and relaxing effect. For women with anxiety who are carrying a lot of physical and emotional tension, blue lessens the fight-or-flight response. Blue also calms such physiological functions as pulse rate, breathing, and perspiration, and relaxes the mood. If you experience chronic fatigue and are tense, anxious, or irritable, or carry a lot of muscle tension, the first exercise will be very helpful.

The second exercise uses the color red, which can benefit women who have fatigue due to chronic anxiety and upset. Red stimulates all the endocrine glands, including the pituitary and adrenal glands. It heightens senses such as smell and taste. Emotionally, red is linked to vitality and high energy states. Even though the color red can speed up autonomic nervous system function, women with anxiety-related fatigue can benefit from visualizing this color. I often do the red visualization when I am tired and need a pick-me-up. You may find that you are attracted to the color in one exercise more than another. Use the exercise with the color that appeals to you the most.

The last two exercises use positive visualizations to engender feelings of love and connection to God, the Divine Source of love, peace, joy and compassion. These two exercises use the incredible power of visualization to help eliminate feelings of anxiety and stress and replace them with positive, nurturing and life-enhancing emotions.

The visualization on love will greatly enhance your mood and assist you in eliminating unwanted emotions like fear, stress and anxiety by helping you to nurture and lovingly care for yourself. The visualization on Divine healing water was created to reinforce your connection to God, our Creator.

These are two of my favorite exercises for their great benefits of elevating our thoughts and feelings in a positive way. I always feel very loving, peaceful and calm when I do them myself.

### Exercise 11: Tension Release Through Color

- Sit or lie in a comfortable position, your arms resting at your sides. As you take a deep breath, visualize that the earth below you is filled with the color blue. Now imagine that you are opening up energy centers on the bottom of your feet. As you inhale, visualize the soft blue color filling up your feet. When your feet are completely filled with the color blue, then bring the color up through your ankles, legs, pelvis, and lower back.

- Each time you exhale, see the blue color leaving through your lungs, carrying any tension and stress with it. See the tension dissolve into the air.

- Continue to inhale the blue color into your abdomen, chest, shoulders, arms, neck, and head. Exhale the blue slowly out of your lungs. Repeat this entire process five times and then relax for a few minutes.

*Exercise 12: Energizing Through Color*

- Sit or lie in a comfortable position, your arms resting easily at your sides. As you take a deep breath, visualize a big balloon above your head filled with a bright red healing energy. Imagine that you pop this balloon so all the bright red energy is released.

- As you inhale, see the bright red color filling up your head. It fills up your brain, your face, and the bones of your skull. Let the bright red color pour in until your head is ready to overflow with color. Then let the red color flow into your neck, shoulders, arms, and chest. As you exhale, breathe the red color out of your lungs, taking any tiredness and fatigue with it. Breathe any feeling of fatigue out of your body.

- As you inhale, continue to bring the bright, energizing red color into your abdomen, pelvis, lower back, legs, and feet until your whole body is filled with red. Exhale the red color out of your lungs, continuing to release any feeling of fatigue. Repeat this process five times. At the end of this exercise, you should feel more energized and vibrant. Your mental energy should feel more vitalized and clear.

*Exercise 13: Loving Yourself*

- To do this visualization, find a quiet spot where you can sit or lie comfortably. As you take a deep breath, focus on the area of your heart (located just to the left of the center of your chest).

- As you inhale and exhale slowly and deeply, close your eyes and envision your heart as a luminous, emerald-green jewel glowing with love and sending out brilliant light from behind your breastbone, where your heart resides.

- As you breathe slowly, begin to fill your heart with love. Feel the area surrounding your heart soften and expand as you fill it with loving and peaceful energy.

- Next, send love and appreciation to every part of your body, even the parts that you are concerned about or feel are less than lovable. They are all parts or you and worthy of the deepest love and caring.

- Breathe love and appreciation into your head, neck, shoulders, chest and down your arms and hands. Send this loving and healing breathe next into your abdomen, hips, legs and feet.

- Continue loving and appreciating yourself until you feel your entire body overflowing with love.

- Now gently open your eyes and slowly begin to move around again. Enjoy the feelings of love, peace and gratitude you have created.

## Exercise 14: Divine Healing Water

- Sit or lie in a comfortable position, with your arms resting gently by your sides.

- Now, close your eyes and breathe deeply. Let your breathing be slow and relaxed.

- Visualize a river of living water flowing gently through you. This is Divine healing water, full of God's light and love.

  Feel this healing water flow into every cell of your body, cleansing you of all cares and worries, bringing you the deepest peace.

- Let this healing water flow through your head, renewing your mind and then moving into your neck and shoulders. As it moves through you, it carries away any tension and tightness.

- Then feel this Divine water flow gently into your chest and down your arms and hands, and then into your abdomen, bringing with it healing and life energy.

- Next, let this water move into your hips and pelvis and down into your legs and feet.

- As this Divine water leaves your body, all darkness is disappearing and is being replaced by light, love and happiness.

- Let this Divine healing water flow through you as long as you would like it to. Continue this process until you feel totally at peace and deeply relaxed.

## Affirmations

The following two exercises give you healthful affirmations that are very positive and life-affirming. I have shared these with many patients who have found them to be helpful in repatterning their mind and beliefs in a much more positive and joyful way. Anxiety, stress and worry symptoms are due to a complex interplay between the mind and body. Your state of emotional and physical health is determined in part by the thousands of mental messages you send yourself each day with your thoughts.

For example, if fear of public places triggers your anxiety symptoms, the mind will send a constant stream of messages to you reinforcing your beliefs about the dangers and mishaps that can occur in public places. The fright triggers muscle tension and shallow breathing. Similarly, if you constantly criticize the way you look; your lack of self-love may be reflected in your body. For example, your shoulders will slump and you may have a dull and lackluster countenance.

Affirmations provide a method to change these negative belief systems to thoughts that reinforce the positives in your life. They uplift your thinking to appreciation and gratitude for all that you have in your life and to seeing yourself for the special and wonderful woman that you are. The positive statements contained in affirmations replace the anxiety-inducing messages with thoughts that make you feel good about yourself and your life. The first affirmation exercise gives you a series of statements to promote a sense of emotional and physical health and well-being. Using these affirmations can help create feelings of emotional peace and positivity by changing your negative beliefs about your body and health into positive beliefs.

The second affirmation exercise helps promote self-esteem and self-confidence and also helps to reduce anxiety. Many women with high anxiety lose their self-confidence and feel depressed and defeated by their condition. They feel frustrated and somehow at fault for not finding a solution. Repeat each affirmation to yourself, write them in a journal or say them out loud. You can use either or both exercises on a regular basis to promote healthful, positive thought patterns.

## *Exercise 13: Positive Mind-Body Affirmations*

- I handle stress and tension appropriately and effectively.
- My mood is calm and relaxed.
- I can cope well and get on with my life during times of stress.
- I think thoughts that uplift and nurture me.
- I enjoy thinking positive thoughts that make me feel good about myself and my life.
- I deserve to feel good right now.
- I feel peaceful and calm.
- My breathing is slow and calm.
- My muscles are relaxed and comfortable.
- I feel grounded and fully present.
- I can effectively handle any situation that comes my way
- I create positive solutions for any challenges in my life.
- I am confident and proud of my ability to manage stress in a calm and peaceful way that creates positive outcomes.
- I am thankful for all the positive things in my life.

## Exercise 14: Self-Esteem Affirmations

- I am filled with energy, vitality, and self-confidence.
- I am pleased with how well I handle my emotional needs.
- I know how to manage my daily schedule to promote my emotional and physical well-being.
- I listen to my body's needs and regulate my activity level to take care of those needs.
- I love and honor my body.
- I fill my mind with positive and self-nourishing thoughts.
- I am a wonderful and worthy person.
- I deserve health, vitality, and peace of mind.
- I have total confidence in my ability to heal myself.
- I am full of energy and vitality.
- The world around me is full of radiant beauty and abundance.
- I am attracted only to those people and situations that support and nurture me.
- I appreciate the positive people and situations that are currently in my life.
- I love and honor myself.
- I enjoy my positive thoughts and feelings.

## More Stress Reduction Techniques for Anxiety

The rest of this chapter contains additional techniques useful for relief of anxiety and relaxation of tight and tense muscles. These methods induce deep emotional relaxation. Try them for a delightful experience.

### Hydrotherapy

For centuries, people have used warm water as a way to calm moods and relax muscles. You can have your own "spa" at home by adding relaxing ingredients to the bath water. I have found the following formula to be extremely useful in relieving muscle pain and tension.

*Alkaline Bath.* Run a tub of warm water. Add one cup of sea salt and one cup of sodium bicarbonate (baking soda) to the tub. You can also add a few drops of relaxing essential oils like lavender and rose water. This is a highly alkaline mixture and I recommend using it once or twice a month. I've found it helpful in reducing cramps and calming anxiety and irritability. Soak for 20 minutes.

You will feel very relaxed after this bath. You may want to use it at night before going to sleep. You will probably wake up feeling refreshed and energized the following day.

Heat of any kind also helps to release muscle tension. Many women find that saunas and baths also help to calm their moods. Heat will increase your menstrual flow, so keep the water a little cooler if heavy flow is a problem.

### Sound

Music can have a tremendously relaxing effect on our minds and bodies. For women with anxiety and nervous tension, I recommend slow, quiet music—classical music is particularly good. This type of music can have a pronounced beneficial effect on your physiological functions. It can slow your pulse and heart rate, lower your blood pressure, and decrease your levels of stress hormones. It promotes peace and relaxation and helps to induce sleep.

Nature sounds, such as ocean waves and rainfall, can also promote a sense of peace and relaxation. I have patients who keep tapes of nature sounds in their cars and at home for use when they feel more stressed. Play relaxing music often when you are aware of increased emotional and physical tension.

## *Massage*

Massage can be extremely therapeutic for women who feel anxious. Gentle touching either by a trained massage therapist, your relationship partner, or even yourself can be very relaxing. Tension usually fades away relatively quickly with gentle, relaxed touching. The kneading and stroking movement of a good massage relaxes tight muscles and improves circulation. During times of stress, if you can afford to do so, I recommend treating yourself to a professional massage. Otherwise, trade with a friend or partner. There are many books available that instruct people how to do a relaxing massage.

## Putting Your Stress Reduction Program Together

This chapter has introduced you to many different ways to reduce anxiety and stress and make each day calm and peaceful. You can try each exercise or do the ones that appeal to you the most. You will find the combination that works best for you. Over time, they will help to relieve anxiety and stress and repattern your emotional responses. These exercises will help to eliminate negative feelings and beliefs while changing them into positive, self-nurturing new ones. Your feelings of anxiety should diminish greatly and your ability to cope with stress will improve tremendously with regular practice.

# 10

## Breathing Exercises for Peace and Relaxation

I love doing breathing exercises for their wonderful calming and relaxing benefits! Focusing on your breathing and taking slow, deep breaths are among the best ways to combat the emotional and physical symptoms of anxiety and stress. Practicing the art of deep breathing can have a major beneficial impact on every aspect of your health and well-being, as well as reducing feelings of tension and upset. They will also help to generate a feeling of internal peace and calm, as well as relax and loosen your muscles.

When you are breathing slowly and deeply, you take in large amounts of oxygen from the environment. This oxygen is taken into your circulation where it binds to the red blood cells as it travels through the arteries and veins. Oxygen allows the cells to produce and utilize energy and to help remove waste products through the production of carbon dioxide. These waste products are cleared through exhalation by the lungs. Thus, the whole body needs optimal levels of oxygen for its normal cycle of building, repair, and elimination.

When you are in emotional distress, oxygen levels decrease. Breathing tends to become jagged, erratic, and shallow. You may find yourself breathing too fast or you may even stop breathing altogether and hold your breath for prolonged periods of time without realizing it.  This can actually worsen your symptoms of anxiety.

Anxious breathing is often linked to other unhealthy physiological reactions that reflect your body's state of stress. When you are upset and emotionally stressed, you tend to tense and tighten your muscles, constrict blood flow, elevate your pulse rate and heartbeat, and stimulate the output of stressful chemicals from your glands. Waste products such as carbon dioxide and lactic acid also accumulate in your muscles and other tissues.

Therapeutic breathing exercises provide a way to break this pattern and help the mind and body return to a peaceful equilibrium. It is important to do the breathing exercises in a slow and regular manner. First, find a comfortable position. You can either do the exercises lying on your back or sitting upright in a chair or on a mat. Be sure to uncross your arms and legs, and keep your back straight.

### Exercise 1: Deep Abdominal Breathing

Deep, slow abdominal breathing is a very important technique for the relief of anxiety and stress. It also improves energy and vitality. Abdominal breathing brings adequate oxygen, the fuel for metabolic activity, to all tissues of the body. In contrast, rapid, shallow breathing decreases oxygen supply and keeps you nervous and tense. Deep breathing helps to relax the entire body and strengthens muscles in the chest and abdomen. Do this exercise for 3 to 5 minutes.

- Lie flat on your back with your knees pulled up or sit upright in a chair in a relaxed manner. Keep your feet slightly apart. Try to breathe in and out through your nose.

- Inhale deeply. As you breathe in, allow your stomach to relax so the air flows into your abdomen. Your stomach should balloon out as you breathe in. Visualize your lungs filling up with air so that your chest swells out.

- Imagine that the air you breathe is filling your body with energy.

- Exhale deeply. As you breathe out, let your stomach and chest collapse. Imagine the air being pushed out, first from your abdomen and then from your lungs.

## *Exercise 2: Peaceful, Slow Breathing*

Breathing slowly and peacefully can decrease anxiety and promote a sense of inner calm. Such breathing helps our mind to slow down and our emotions to become happier and more harmonious. Life feels good. When we are calm, we make better decisions and relate to those around us in a healthier way. Breathing slowly can also calm our physical responses by helping to balance autonomic nervous system function. By slowing down our breathing, we slow down our other physiologic responses. Our muscles relax and our blood vessels dilate; a state of equilibrium is restored.

- Lie flat on your back with your knees pulled up. Keep your feet slightly apart. Try to breathe in and out through your nose.

- Inhale deeply. As you breathe in, allow your stomach to relax so that the air flows into your abdomen. Let your stomach balloon out as you breathe in. Visualize the lowest parts of your lungs filling up with air.

- Imagine that the air you are breathing in is filled with peace and calm; a sensation of peacefulness and calm is filling every cell of your body; your whole body feels warm and relaxed as you breathe in this air. Now, exhale deeply. As you breathe out, imagine the air being pushed out from the bottom of your lungs to the top.

- Repeat this sequence until your entire body feels relaxed and your breathing is slow and regular.

## *Exercise 3: Color Breathing with Golden Light*

Color breathing has traditionally been used to heal the mind and body and strengthen the body's energy field. Some people are able to see this energy field as light or colors emanating from the body.

When a person is calm, relaxed and healthy, the energy field appears radiant and full of colors. The colors tend to be bright and harmonious. When we are feeling anxious or tense, we lose light and color. Our energy field looks more discordant and jagged, and often the colors change to duller, more muddied colors.

Color breathing is a technique that can help strengthen and heal the energy field as well as calm the mind and body. As you breathe in the healing colors, you often begin to relax and feel more peaceful. Anxiety and tension are replaced by a sensation of lightness and calm.

- Sit or lie in a comfortable position.

- Imagine beautiful golden energy surrounding you. As you take a deep breath, inhale the golden energy and visualize it flowing through your body—a healing energy that warms and relaxes you.

- Hold the inhalation as long as it is comfortable. Let this golden energy dissolve all your anxiety and tension.

- Then, as you exhale this energy out through your lungs, visualize all of your tension and stress leaving your body, dissolving and disappearing.

- Repeat this process as many times as needed until a feeling of peace and calm replaces any anxiety and stress that you may be holding.

## Exercise 4: Emotional Healing Breath

I have seen during my years of medical practice that our negative feelings and belief systems are major triggers of anxiety, nervous tension, and even physical illness. This exercise again uses color breathing. This time you will using healing light to help you release negative feelings such as chronic anger, hurt, or other upsets you may be harboring.

The more time you spend cleansing and releasing old negative emotional patterns, the less impact they will have on your moods and your life. This is a great breathing exercise to do if you are feeling upset, angry, hurt or fearful. It will help you feel more positive, peaceful and centered.

- Lie flat on your back with your knees pulled up or sit upright in a comfortable position. Keep your feet slightly apart. Breathe in and out through your nose.

- Inhale deeply and see yourself enveloped in a soft white light. Breathe this light into every cell of your body. This is a cleansing light and you can visualize it washing away fear, anger, anxiety, and any other negative feelings that you may be experiencing.

- As you exhale, feel the light washing these emotions away, dissolving them, replacing them with positive feelings of peace, joy and love.

- Repeat this exercise until you feel emotionally peaceful and clear.

## *Exercise 5: Muscle Tension Release Breathing*

I want to share with you a wonderful exercise that will help you to get in touch with and release any muscle tension and tightness and bring your body back into a state of healthy balance. Often when you are anxious and upset, you may unconsciously tense up muscles throughout the entire body. The neck, shoulders, lower back, hips and other areas of the body are particularly vulnerable.

Muscle tension often occurs in response to the stresses of the day or from sitting in one position for hours at the desk or computer and even after doing vigorous exercise. After doing this meditation, you will feel more peaceful and relaxed!

- Sit or lie in a comfortable position. Allow your arms to rest at your sides, palms down and inhale and exhale slowly and deeply.

- Become aware of your feet, ankles, and legs. Notice if these parts of your body have any muscle tension or tightness. Breathe into that part of your body until you feel it relax.

- Next, move your awareness into your hips, pelvis, and lower back. Note any tension there. Breathe into your hips and pelvis until you feel them relax. Release any emotional stress as you breathe in and out.

- Focus on your abdomen and chest. Notice any tension or tightness located in this area and let it drop away as you breathe in and out. Continue to breathe into this area until your chest and abdomen feel relaxed.

- Finally, focus on your head, neck, arms, and hands. Note any tension in this area and release it. With your breathing, release any negative emotions blocked in this area until you feel peaceful and calm.

- When you have finished releasing tension throughout the body, continue deep breathing and relaxing for another minute or two. At the end of this exercise, you should feel lighter, relaxed and more energized.

*Exercise 6: Upper Body Muscle Release*

This exercise will help you focus on any tension that you are carrying in your upper body. Relaxing and releasing the muscles in your neck and shoulders will help release muscle tension in your entire body. To get in touch with any muscle tension that you may be carrying, use this exercise while walking or doing sports or desk work.

- Sit upright in a chair. Be sure you are in a comfortable position. Keep your feet slightly apart. Try to breathe in and out through your nose.

- Inhale and exhale deeply. As you breathe, let your head move from side to side. Keep your shoulders down and try to touch your ear to your shoulder. As you do this movement, imagine that your neck is made out of putty and that it allows your head to move in a supple, relaxed movement from the left to the right.

- Now inhale and pull your shoulders up towards your ears. Hold your breath and keep your shoulders in a hunched position. Exhale and let your shoulders drop back into a relaxed, comfortable position. Repeat this several times.

- Inhale and exhale deeply as you roll your shoulders forward. Make a large, slow, circular motion with your shoulders. Then roll your shoulders back slowly, again inhaling and exhaling. Repeat this sequence several times.

- Inhale and exhale deeply, keeping the rest of your body still and relaxed. Repeat this several times.

## Exercise 7: Divine Healing Breath

This is one of my favorite and most inspirational breathing and meditation exercises. I always feel uplifted when I do this exercise. It is a beautiful meditation on filling yourself with the Divine light and love of God. This meditation will also help you release any tension or negativity from your mind and fill you with wonderful feelings of peace and joy.

- Begin the meditation by finding a quiet place. It can be a peaceful room in your house or office or even a beautiful spot in your backyard. Then, sit or lie in a comfortable position, with your arms resting gently by your sides.

- Close your eyes and breathe deeply. Let your breathing be slow and relaxed. Visualize yourself as a flower in the sun, opening yourself to God's light and love. Feel this Divine light surrounding you and enfolding you, filling every cell of your body with love.

- As this light fills and nurtures you, you are being cleansed of all cares and worries. This Divine light is dispelling all darkness as it gently and lovingly restores you to a state of health, balance and peace.

- Visualize this Divine light, bringing brightness and clarity into your mind, your head and then your neck and shoulders. As it moves through you, it carries away any tension and tightness.

- As you continue to breathe deeply and slowly, feel the warmth of this light as it moves into your chest and down your arms and hands, and then into your abdomen, bringing with it healing and protection.

- Next, let this Divine light move into your hips and pelvis and finally down into your legs and feet.

- Let this Divine light move through you as long as you would like it to. Continue this process until you feel totally at peace and deeply relaxed.

- Know that God is always with you, caring for you and loving you always.

## Exercise 8: Glandular Breathing

This exercise helps stimulate and energize your endocrine glands through the use of color breathing. When you direct your breath into the endocrine glands and visualize them being stimulated by the color, the glands are, in fact, stimulated in a beneficial way. The use of color breathing expands the electromagnetic field of the endocrine glands. In this exercise, the color red is used; in research studies, red light has been shown to stimulate both the endocrine and immune functions.

- Sit upright in a chair, your arms at your sides, palms up. Visualize a soft cloud or energy field filled with the color red above your head. It is a bright, vibrant tone of red that sparkles with energy.

- As you inhale deeply, see the red energy flowing into your head and concentrating in the hypothalamus, a gland located near the center of the brain. You can visualize the area of this endocrine gland by focusing the red energy in the area between your eyes (sometimes called "the third eye" area). As the hypothalamus begins to overflow with color, exhale and let the red energy flow out of your lungs, filling the air around you.

- As you inhale again, breathe the bright red color into your pituitary, an important endocrine gland located in your brain, right below the hypothalamus. Fill the pituitary with this color until it overflows. Then exhale deeply releasing any excess red energy.

- As you continue to inhale the bright red color, let it flow into your thyroid gland, located at the base of your neck, then into your thymus gland, located in the middle of your chest. Finally, let the color energize your adrenal glands, located in the middle of your back above the kidneys, and finally your ovaries, located in the pelvis. As you fill up each endocrine gland with red energy, continue to release any excess energy into the air around you as you exhale.

- When you finish this exercise, relax for a few minutes. You should feel energized and bright, yet peaceful and calm at the same time.

Anxiety and nervous tension often deplete endocrine gland function. If your endocrine glands are overly stressed, you may feel anxious and tired. You may also be prone to imbalances like PMS, menopause symptoms, hypoglycemia, and thyroid disease. In addition, you may also be more likely to develop infections like colds and flu, because the endocrine glands help regulate the immune function.

## Putting Your Breathing Exercise Program Together

In this chapter, I have shared with you many wonderful and enjoyable breathing exercises to help reduce anxiety and tension as well as support improved health and more peace and joy. You may want to try each exercise once or choose those that most appeal to you. I recommend practicing breathing exercises on a regular basis for their great anxiety and stress reducing benefits. These exercises can help you even if you practice them only a few minutes each day. Over time, healthy breathing habits will become automatic and will also greatly benefit your general health.

# 11

## Physical Exercises

Exercise is an important part of your anxiety and stress reduction program. The discharge of physical and emotional tension that accompanies a vigorous session of exercise directly and immediately reduces anxiety and stress. In addition, the long-term physiological benefits of exercise build up your resistance to stress and promote beneficial psychological changes. Let us look at how exercise produces these changes in the body and mind.

### The Benefits of Exercise

*Exercise Improves Resistance to and Relief of Anxiety Episodes*

When women have excessive anxiety and tension due to lifestyle stress or emotional problems, the sympathetic nervous system is easily tripped, producing the fight-or-flight response. The same is true for women who are in a state of hormonal or physiological imbalance caused by PMS, menopause, hypoglycemia, overactivity of the thyroid, or mitral valve prolapse.

The problem for many women who have chronic anxiety and tension is that their sympathetic nervous system is always in a state of readiness to a crisis. This puts them in a constant state of tension, causing them to react to small stresses the same way they react to real emergencies. Their adrenal glands increase their output of adrenaline and cortisone, and their thyroid gland pumps out thyroxin (the thyroid hormone), adjusting the body chemistry to meet the crisis. Their heart speeds up, their pulses race, and their neck and shoulder muscles tense, as do muscles in other parts of the body.

These tight and tense muscles have decreased blood flow and oxygenation. Waste products such as excessive carbon dioxide accumulate in this physical environment and can further worsen fight-or-flight symptoms. In addition, stress causes breathing to become rapid and shallow. Less oxygen is taken in through respiration, which further decreases the oxygen available to the muscles and internal organs.

The tension that accumulates in the body to meet this "emergency" must then be discharged. Often it is discharged emotionally by triggering a panic attack or emotional meltdown that is physically and emotionally draining. Some women deal with this fight-or-flight reaction by discharging their anxiety through eating harmful food, alcohol, or cigarette addictions. Overeating often becomes a way of diffusing tension. The habitual indulgence in addictive behavior is additionally harmful to the body. If you have a condition like PMS, you may find that you are irritable with your children or being rude and abrupt with people at work.

Physical exercise, particularly moderate aerobic types that helps to slow down and discharge the fight-or-flight tension is very beneficial. Exercise improves oxygenation and blood circulation to tight muscles and devitalized organ systems. By improving circulation, exercise facilitates proper nutrient flow throughout the body. Removal of waste products such as carbon dioxide, lactic acid, and other products of metabolism become more efficient. The acidity or pH of the blood is lowered to an optimal range, and the production of energy by the cells becomes more efficient. This is important since optimal energy production is needed to run the body's many chemical and physiological functions.

In contrast, I do not recommend that women with anxiety do intense anaerobic types of exercise like fast running or jogging or heavy weight lifting since these types of exercise actually intensify the physiological imbalances caused by anxiety and stress. With anxiety and panic attacks, you need to slow down and relax, not make your body more tense. That is why relaxed walking, hiking, bike riding, swimming, playing golf, gardening and other types of more mellow and relaxing exercises are actually beneficial in reducing the stress response if you tend towards anxiety. You can hike and bike long distances but it is more beneficial for your stress response to do it in a slower paced manner.

With regular moderate aerobic exercise, the heart muscle also works more efficiently. As the heart becomes conditioned, it is able to pump more blood with each stroke. Thus, it can circulate the same volume of blood with fewer strokes and doesn't have to work as hard. Once an exercise program is initiated, the resting heart rate soon slows down quite markedly. Research studies show that the beneficial changes can occur rapidly, often within several months.

A lower resting heart rate means more than increased strength and stamina. A healthier heart also reacts less dramatically during episodes of anxiety and stress. When anxiety causes the adrenal glands to pump out stressor hormones, a conditioned heart will not experience a significant rise in the heart rate. In a stressful situation, a fit person may have only a slight rise in heart rate, while a sedentary person may experience a terrifying pounding of the heart and shortness of breath. Not only does a fit woman tend to stay calmer and more in control of her emotions during a taxing situation, but also in periods of extreme stress, her good physical conditioning may help prevent a heart attack and thereby save her life.

### Exercise Improves Brain Function

Besides improving cardiovascular function, regular exercise also reduces anxiety by improving brain function. Healthy brain function is necessary to decrease nervous tension and reduce the tendency toward panic episodes and phobias. After exercising, you will feel more peaceful, calmer, and even happier. You will certainly feel more refreshed and energized.

How does exercise promote such striking emotional changes? Exercise brings better oxygenation and circulation to the brain and nerves by opening up and dilating blood vessels of the head and brain. Thus, more nutrients can flow into, and more waste products can be removed from, this vital system. In fact, 20 percent of the blood flow from the heart goes directly to the brain. The brain also utilizes a large share (again, 20 percent) of the body's nutrients and energy.

Research studies done on adults who exercise compared with similar groups who are sedentary show striking differences in a variety of mental functions. Adults engaged in an active exercise program have better concentration, and clearer and quicker thinking and problem solving. In addition, reaction time and short-term memory improve.

Not only does regular exercise induce functional improvements in the brain, it also dramatically alters brain chemistry in a positive way through the increased production of beta-endorphins. Beta-endorphins, are chemicals released from the pituitary glands, which act as natural opiates. They are chemically similar to the pain reliever morphine, but 200 times more potent. Endorphins have a dramatic effect on mood. When levels in the body are high, they improve a woman's general sense of well-being. Beta-endorphin levels increase after ovulation, during the early part of the second half of the menstrual cycle (called the luteal phase by physicians).

As menstruation approaches, beta-endorphin levels can begin to fall. In fact, some PMS researchers believe that the drop in beta-endorphins may be responsible for the emotional symptoms of PMS such as anxiety, irritability, and mood swings. These are the predominant symptoms in more than 80 percent of women with PMS.

Exercise helps reduce anxiety and nervous tension by increasing the production of beta-endorphins. Some women who exercise regularly report feelings of elation, euphoria, and even bliss. Aerobic exercise may even help cushion the premenstrual fall in beta-endorphins and thereby reduce PMS-related anxiety.

### Exercise Improves Psychological Function

Since the beta-endorphins tend to elevate mood and promote well-being, exercise can also be an effective antidote for depression. While the standard treatment for depression is psychotherapy and antidepressant medication, a number of interesting chemical studies have shown that exercise significantly helps relieve moderate depression.

Psychotherapists who treat women for emotional disorders are aware that these two conditions, anxiety and depression, frequently coexist. Even with health issues like PMS and menopause, which are primarily due to a variety of hormonal and chemical imbalances (rather than emotional causes), anxiety and depression often both occur. Women with these problems will complain that their mood vacillates between nervous or irritable and sad and depressed. Exercise can be a powerful antidote for problems on both ends of the emotional spectrum.

Women who are anxious and nervous often have difficulty sleeping at night. They may lie in bed for two to three hours, their minds busy with "chatter" and self-talk. Often this self-talk includes fearful thoughts and worries about stressful life situations or even imagined concerns. Some women have difficulty sleeping when their anxiety is mixed with strong anger, hostility, and upset toward a person or difficult situation. I have had anxious patients tell me that they have tried strong sleeping medications or alcoholic beverages to induce sleep; however, upset feelings can override the sedative effects of the medication or alcohol. This can lead to drug and alcohol abuse as women increase their intake in an effort to shut off their disturbing thoughts and feelings at night.

Exercise can help to reduce insomnia by working off nervous energy and diffusing the fight-or-flight response. After exercise, both the body and mind are calmer. It is often easier for women to relax and sleep soundly when they have included a session of physical activity in their daily schedule. Exercise should not, however, be done late in the day by women suffering from insomnia, since the energizing effects of the exercise are not desirable late at night. It is better to exercise earlier in the day if better sleep quality is one of your main goals.

Other psychological benefits can come from the act of exercising itself. Regular exercise demands discipline and a willingness to overcome resistance and inertia. Anxious and stressed women often feel as if their life is out of control or their life's structure is falling apart. This is particularly true for women who have frequent panic attacks, are crippled by phobias, or suffer from a constant high level of anxiety and nervousness.

Choosing specific times to exercise and then exercising on a regular basis provides structure and discipline. A woman who begins a session of walking, bike riding, swimming or golf feeling anxious will often find her mind focusing on the activity itself or the attractive surroundings, such as a golf course or swimming area. As the session progresses, tension will fade away.

Also, since many forms of exercise or sport do require a level of skill mastery, regular physical activity gives a tremendous boost of self-confidence in women who feel they have no control over their emotions. Mastery of a physical skill provides the blueprint for handling emotional upsets more effectively. This allows you to handle your problems with more self-esteem, an improved self-image, and greater coping skills.

Engaging in regular exercise is also a good, healthful habit. It is a great substitute for more harmful ways of dealing with stress such as overeating, alcohol abuse, or combative behavior. Exercising regularly, three to five times a week, is a positive habit that has many beneficial effects on health.

### Exercise Improves Physiological Functions

Exercise can also have a beneficial effect on anxiety due to physiological factors. For instance, exercise helps to reduce stress symptoms due to hypoglycemia or PMS-related sugar cravings by stabilizing the blood sugar level. Along with diet, exercise can help reduce the tendency toward such common hypoglycemia symptoms such as anxiety, jitteriness, inability to concentrate, and dizziness. Exercise helps iron out the roller coaster blood sugar highs and lows from which women with hypoglycemia suffer.

Exercise also has a beneficial effect on our intake and processing of food. It reduces excessive cravings for food, both for women with food addictions and for women with PMS who tend to overeat high stress foods in the week or two prior to the onset of menstruation. This curbing of excessive appetite and overeating improves our ability to lose and maintain a healthy weight.

Exercise also improves the body's ability to burn calories more rapidly and efficiently. This provides an additional boost to weight loss. Exercise benefits the general health of many other systems, too. Elimination through the bowels and kidneys is improved, which also helps to regulate weight and water balance. Constipation is less likely to be a problem in active women. It reduces the tendency have to anxiety-related digestive symptoms such as abdominal cramping, discomfort and bloating.

In fact, I have had patients with stress-related intestinal symptoms report symptom relief immediately following exercise sessions. Exercise also helps reduce blood pressure levels, which takes stress off the heart and contributes to a reduction of heart attack risk. In summary, exercise benefits the entire body and promotes good health.

## Benefits of Exercise

*Improves resistance to and relief of anxiety episodes*
- Reduces the fight-or-flight response
- Promotes cardiovascular resistance to stress
- Decreases skeletal muscle tension
- Reduces pent-up aggression and frustration
- Promotes a feeling of calm and peace

*Improves brain function*
- Promotes better oxygenation and blood circulation to the brain
- Increases output of beta endorphins
- Improves concentration, problem solving, reaction time, and short-term memory

*Improves psychological functions*
- Decreases anxiety and nervous tension
- Produces a sense of well-being and even elation
- Reduces depression
- Reduces insomnia
- Improves sense of mastery and self-confidence
- Promotes development of beneficial habits
- Helps decrease harmful addictive behavior

*Improves physiological functions*
- Stabilizes blood sugar level
- Reduces food craving
- Helps weight loss and maintenance
- Improves elimination through the bowels and kidneys
- Improves digestive functions
- Reduces blood pressure

## Building Your Exercise Program

### *Evaluating Your Fitness Level*

If you are currently making the transition from a sedentary lifestyle to a regular exercise program, it is a good idea to evaluate your level of fitness. It is important to know if you have any undiagnosed medical problems that could affect your level of activity. These would include problems like undiagnosed thyroid disease and hypoglycemia, which can trigger anxiety symptoms in connection with exercise. I have had patients with thyroid imbalance, for example, who felt more anxious and short of breath when exercising, because their excessive levels of thyroid hormone were elevating their heart and pulse rates to unhealthy levels during times of increased activity. It is important to consult with a physician or other caregiver to rule out any physical causes for your tendency towards anxiety or panic episodes.

If you have not already done so, I recommend that you fill out the workbook section questionnaires on your current exercise habits, patterns of muscle tension, and symptoms of lack of physical fitness. If you find that you have chronic muscle tension or feel out-of-breath after walking up a flight of stairs, you may actually have an underlying problem like anemia (low red blood cell count), which can often go undiagnosed if the symptoms are merely due to living a sedentary lifestyle.

As mentioned in chapter 3 on the diagnosis of anxiety, I suggest that you share your responses to these questionnaires with your health care provider because they may offer valuable clues to help discover a medical problem that hasn't yet been diagnosed. In addition, be sure to let your physician know if you have any previously diagnosed problems such as mitral valve prolapse, which can also trigger anxiety-like episodes.

Your physician should check your heart, lungs, pulse rate, and other physical parameters to evaluate your exercise fitness. Blood and urine tests are also frequently ordered. Depending on the age of the woman, blood sugar, thyroid, and menopause blood tests are frequently used when screening for anxiety. If you don't understand any terms or tests used, ask your physician for more information. If you are informed and knowledgeable about any emotional or physical causes underlying your tendency towards feeling anxious or overly stressed, you can do a much better job of creating and participating in your own healing program. Once you have received a clean bill of health or understand any health limitations, you are ready to begin planning your exercise program.

## Choosing an Exercise Program

The type of exercise regimen you choose can vary greatly depending on the goals you wish to accomplish. If your main goal is to relieve anxiety and stress and improve your general health and well-being, then aerobic exercise is best. Examples of aerobic exercise include walking, bicycle riding, swimming, dancing and skating. Aerobic exercise reduces stress, promotes calm and relaxation, and helps reduce the tendency toward insomnia and addictive food and drug behavior. Because it requires active work on the part of your skeletal and heart muscles, it reduces the muscle tension that often accompanies anxiety and improves cardiovascular fitness, oxygenation, and circulation to all the systems of the body, thereby increasing your resistance to stress.

If you find that socializing and playing games with other people helps to reduce nervous tension and stress, then slower-paced sports and games like golf, croquet, and bowling could also provide such relaxation.

For those women whose anxiety and stress symptoms include significant muscle tightness and tension, exercises that promote muscular flexibility, like stretching exercises, can be very helpful. Stretches are performed slowly, along with deep breathing, in a relaxed and careful manner. They are helpful in slowing down an anxious system whose physiology is set on overdrive.

If you want to develop increased muscle strength and stamina through weight lifting I recommend that you use smaller weights rather than doing intense, heavy weight lifting which is anaerobic and oxygen depleting and works against anxiety and stress reduction. Finally, if being outdoors while you discharge anxiety and tension works for you, gardening can be very healing. Bending, lifting, and upper-body movements dissipate anxiety and upset rapidly while you are pulling weeds and digging up the ground for new plantings.

Often, women may combine two or three types of exercise activities to meet a variety of goals. Whatever form of exercise you choose, make sure that it meets the goals of reducing anxiety and stress and promoting an improved sense of calm and well-being.

### Keeping an Exercise Diary

You may want to keep an exercise diary during the first few months of a new exercise program, although this certainly isn't mandatory. I have included a diary form in the workbook section that you can use. You will derive many benefits by keeping an exercise diary. This can help you to determine if your program is providing you with the maximum anxiety-reducing benefits. I recommend that you keep your diary very simple. You can use a notebook, pad of paper or even a sheet of paper to make notes on.

When filling out the diary, the three most important things to record are the dates on which you exercised, the type of exercise you engaged in and, most importantly, your emotional and physical responses to the exercise session. If you skipped a planned session, be sure to record the reason why, such as illness or excessive work demands.

Record both positive and negative responses to your exercise session. When recording your emotional responses, be sure to note if you felt calmer and more relaxed after the session. Also record if your anxiety, panic, or stress symptoms actually increase. This can occur if you are pushing yourself too hard with an exercise program that is too vigorous or demanding. In this case, you may want to reduce the length of time you are exercising, the intensity with which you exercise, or the type of physical activity you're doing.

Increased anxiety can also occur if you get distracted by too much negative self-talk and worry. In this case, you might want to listen to relaxing music while you're exercising, focus on deep breathing, repeat prayers to yourself like the 23rd Psalm of the Bible which is incredibly uplifting and reassuring of God's love for you. You can also pick a visually beautiful place to exercise like a park, hilly terrain or by a body of water like a lake or river. This can help refocus your thoughts on enjoying the environment around you. I discuss this in more detail in the next section on motivating yourself to exercise.

In monitoring your physical responses to exercise, choose such parameters as beneficial changes in muscle tension and pulse rate. Do not continue with an exercise program if it doesn't meet your ultimate goal: reduction of anxiety, stress, and their associated symptoms. With such a wide range of exercises and sports to choose from, you can use your diary to help you determine what mix of physical activities works best for you.

## Motivating Yourself to Exercise

If you encounter mental obstacles to beginning and sticking with a regular exercise program, there are many ways to overcome this resistance. Be sure that you are clear on why you don't want to exercise so that you can address the issues directly. Keeping the exercise diary found in the workbook section should help you pinpoint areas of resistance.

- Make sure you exercise at the time of day that feels most natural. Exercise when you are the least hurried and stressed by your schedule. If your largest amount of free time is in the late afternoon between work and dinner, put aside that time to engage in physical activity.

- Be sure to choose an exercise activity that you enjoy. Don't pick an activity that worsens your anxiety level or that you find boring.

- Exercise in an attractive setting. If you run or walk, pick a setting near you that promotes peace and calm. Walk or run in a park, beach, or even a quiet residential street. Avoid areas with lots of cars and traffic congestion.

- Exercise with a friend. This can be a great help in motivating and encouraging you to begin and stick with an exercise program.

- Use your mind to disconnect from your daily activities. Positive mental exercises can help you to relax before starting physical activity. Many women find that a few minutes of doing visualizations (seeing yourself performing and enjoying the exercise routine) or saying affirmations (positive statements about the benefits of exercise) prepares them for their exercise routine.

- Listen to music while you exercise. Many women find that the exercise period goes by much more quickly and the process is more fun and enjoyable when they listen to music. Be sure to choose music that is mellow and relaxing since it will help improve your mood and relax you further.

### Beginning an Exercise Program for Relief of Anxiety and Stress

Before you begin your exercise program for relief of anxiety and stress, read through the following guidelines. They will help you to perform your exercise program in an optimal manner to promote a deeper sense of calm and relaxation.

These guidelines are particularly good for women who are just beginning an exercise program after leading a sedentary life. They are also helpful for women who have previously been fit and active but stopped exercising because physical exertion seemed to trigger anxiety, panic episodes, or muscle tension.

An exercise program that is too strenuous can leave a woman with anxiety feeling more anxious and uptight than ever. Thus, getting a good start on an exercise program can make a major difference in how well you can stick to and even enjoy your chosen physical activity.

- During the first week or two of your program, build up your exercise level gradually. Limit your initial exercise workouts to short sessions. For example, you might start out exercising every other day for only 10 minutes. Then, increase the length of your sessions gradually in 5-minute increments until you are exercising between 30 and 60 minutes per session.

- Perform the exercise in a relaxed and unhurried manner. Be sure to set aside adequate time so you do not feel rushed. Anytime you feel anxiety, panic, or excessive muscle tension, stop doing the exercise. Then re-evaluate your pace to see if it is too vigorous. Initially you might want to exercise with another person who can provide support if your anxiety symptoms become very severe.

- Wear loose, comfortable clothing. If you are doing stretching, work without socks to give your feet complete freedom of movement and to prevent slipping.

- Try to exercise at least 90 minutes before a meal and wait at least two hours after eating to exercise. Working out before dinner is particularly good since it helps diffuse tensions that have accumulated throughout the day. Evacuate your bowels or bladder before you begin the exercises

- Avoid exercising when you are ill or during times of extreme stress. At such times, the stress-reduction exercises or breathing exercises provided in this book will be more useful.

- Move slowly and carefully when first starting to exercise. This will help promote flexibility of the muscles and prevent injury

- Always rest for a few minutes after finishing a session.

# 12

## Stretches for Relief of Anxiety and Stress

Stretches can help to provide effective relief of anxiety and stress. Always perform them slowly and carefully and accompany the stretches with deep, relaxed breathing. Stretches quiet your mood and promote a deep sense of peace and calm. Unlike fast-paced aerobic exercise, stretches actually slow down your pulse, heart rate, and breathing. This benefits many women with anxiety and tension related to life stress. Stretches provides an oasis of calm in which you can put aside your stress and focus on doing the exercises slowly and on breathing calmly and deeply.

When you practice a series of stretching exercises, you gently stretch every muscle in your body. These exercises relax tense muscles and improve their suppleness and flexibility. They also promote better circulation and oxygenation to tense and contracted areas throughout the body. As a result, general metabolism of the muscles and organ system is improved. Both the stress reduction effects and the physiological effects of stretching benefit all body systems, including digestive and elimination function, the endocrine (glandular) system, the nervous system, and the immune system.

I have included in this chapter a series of stretches that specifically reduce anxiety and stress. Some of these exercises work on the emotions, calming your mood and inducing peace and serenity. Other poses help relieve the physical causes of anxiety and stress, such as PMS and menopause-related problems.

I recommend reading through the exercises first to see which ones apply to your causes of anxiety and stress. You may want to try these exercises first. Or you could try all the exercises initially for the first week or two and see which ones produce the most beneficial results. You can do the stretches three times a week, or even daily if your anxiety and stress symptoms respond well to more frequent practice.

When you begin the anxiety and stress-relief exercises, it is important that you focus your mind and concentrate on the positions. First your mind visualizes how the exercise is to look, then your body follows with the correct execution of the pose. Pay close attention to the initial instructions. Look carefully at the placement of the body in the photographs. If you practice the stretch properly, you are much more likely to have relief of your symptoms.

Move through each pose slowly. This slowness allows you to have greater control over your body movements. You minimize the possibility of injury and maximize the benefit to the particular part of the body that is the focus of the pose. If you practice these stretches regularly in an unhurried fashion, you will also gradually loosen your muscles, ligaments, and joints. You may be surprised at how supple you can become.

If you experience any pain or discomfort, you have probably overreached your current ability and should immediately reduce the amount of the stretching until you can proceed without discomfort. Be careful, as muscular injuries can take quite a while to heal. If you do strain a muscle, apply ice to the injured area for 10 minutes. Use the ice pack two to three times a day for several days. If the pain persists, see your doctor.

Follow the breathing instructions for the exercise. Most important, do not hold your breath. Allow your breath to flow in and out easily and effortlessly.

*Stretch 1*

This exercise is excellent for calming anxiety and stress due to emotional causes, and it will also relieve anxiety and irritability due to PMS and menopause. For women with food addiction episodes or coexisting mitral valve prolapse, it will lessen anxiety. This exercise gently stretches the lower back and is one of the most effective exercises for relieving menstrual cramps.

Sit on your heels. Bring your forehead to the floor, stretching the spine as far over your head as possible.

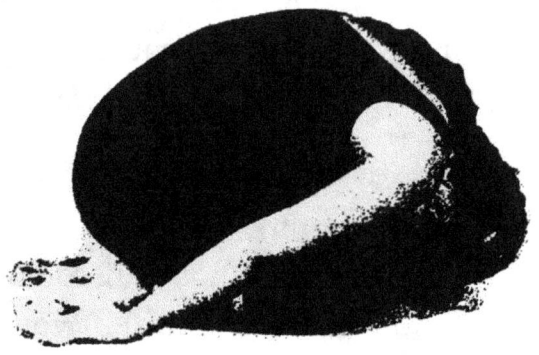

Close your eyes. Hold for as long as comfortable.

*Stretch 2*

This exercise relieves anxiety and stress due to emotional causes, PMS, or menopause. It helps quiet anxiety in women with coexisting food addiction episodes or mitral valve prolapse. It relieves menstrual cramps and low back pain. It also reduces eye tension and swelling in the face.

Lie on your back with a rolled towel placed under your knees. Your arms should be at your sides, palms up.

Close your eyes and relax your whole body. Inhale slowly, breathing from the diaphragm. As you inhale, visualize the energy in the air around you being drawn in through your entire body. Imagine that your body is porous and open like a sponge, so it can draw in this energy to revitalize every cell of your body.

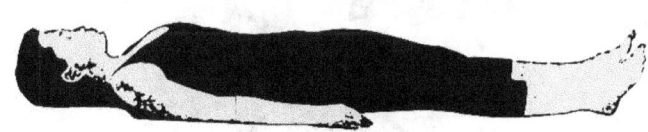

Exhale slowly and deeply, allowing every ounce of tension to drain from your body.

*Stretch 3*

This exercise massages the neck and spine and flexes the vertebral column. It will invigorate and energize you, helping balance your body and mind and reduce fatigue. It also promotes good circulation and relieves low back tension. To enhance the benefits of the exercise, lie flat on your back for a few minutes after doing it.

Lie on your back. Bend and raise your knees to your chest, clasping them with your hands. Hands should be interlocked below knees.

Raise your head toward your knees and gently rock back and forth on your curved spine.

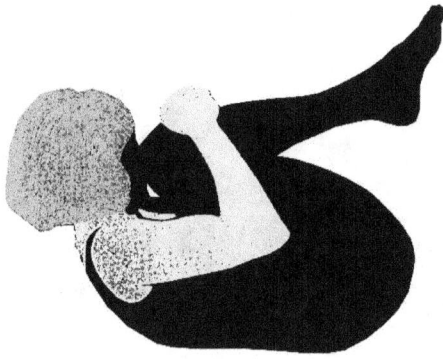

Note the roundness of your back and shoulders. Keep the chin tucked in as you roll back. Avoid rolling back too far on your neck. Rock back and forth 5 to 10 times.

## Stretch 4

This pose reduces anxiety and nervous tension and will help eliminate tension headaches and insomnia. It improves flexibility of the spine, reducing stiffness and back pain.

Lie on your back with your legs bent and your feet together. Place your hands on the sides of both ankles to keep your legs together.

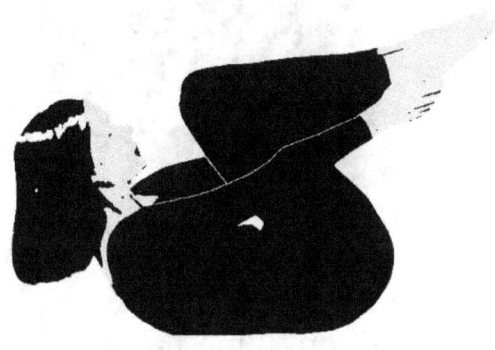

As you inhale, raise your legs up over your head. To make sure that the posture is comfortable, adjust the angle of your legs, bending your knees to apply pressure between the shoulder blades.

Hold this posture for one minute, breathing slowly and deeply.

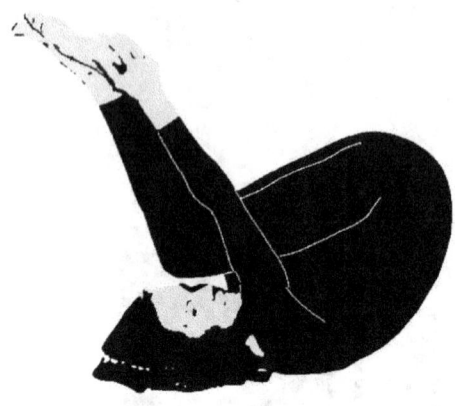

Return to the original position, lying flat on your back with your eyes closed. Relax in this position for several minutes.

## Stretch 5

This exercise calms anxiety and nervousness. It strengthens the back and abdominal muscles and improves blood circulation and oxygenation to the pelvis.

Lie down and press the small of your back into the floor. This permits you to use your abdominal muscles without straining your lower back.

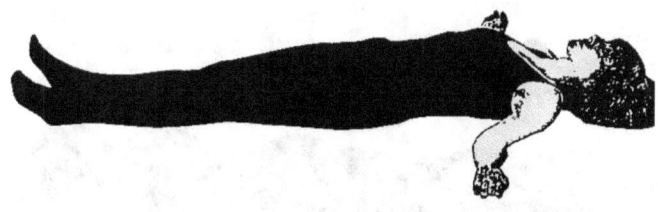

Raise your right leg slowly while breathing in. Let the rest of your body remain relaxed. Move your leg very slowly. Do not move your leg in a jerking manner. Hold for a few breaths.

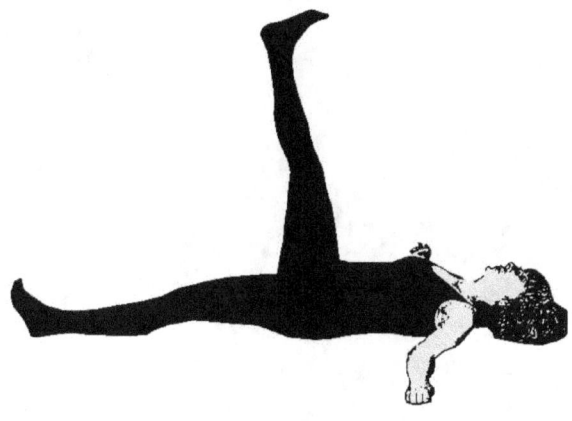

Lower your leg and breathe out. Repeat the same exercise on your left side. Alternate legs; repeat the exercise 5 to 10 times.

## Stretch 6

This exercise reduces anxiety and nervous tension. It also helps to eliminate tension headaches. By stretching the spine, you enhance circulation and improve spinal flexibility.

Lie on your stomach with your chin on the floor and your feet together. Place your palms flat on the floor, underneath your shoulders.

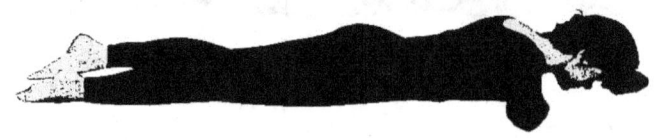

As you inhale, lift your head up, stretching your neck back. Then, raise your chest, using your arms and back muscles.

As you complete the inhalation, arch your body all the way up, keeping your hips on the ground.

As you hold this position, exhale deeply. Then, breathe deeply and slowly, inhaling and exhaling for 30 seconds.

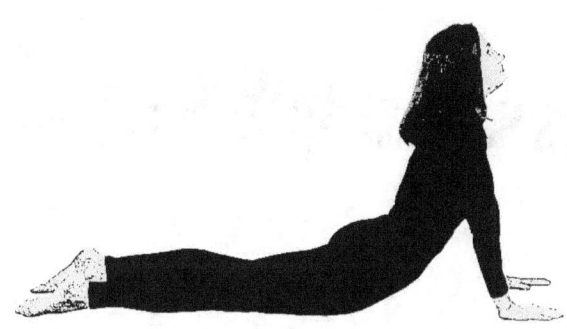

Lower yourself part way, using your arms for support. Holding the body at this angle, breathe deeply for 30 seconds.

Then let your body come all the way down. Relax with your head turned to one side and your arms resting gently on the floor. Close your eyes and relax for several minutes.

## Stretch 7

This exercise helps release overall body tension. It improves circulation and concentration. It strengthens the lower back and abdominal area.

Lie on your stomach with your feet together and your arms lying flat at your sides.

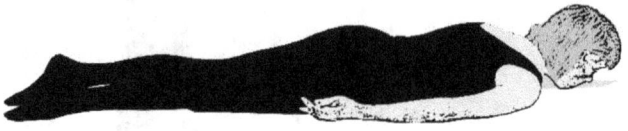

Stretch your arms out straight in front of you on the floor.

As you inhale, arch your back and lift your arms, head, chest and legs off the floor. Hold the pose as long as you can, up to 30 seconds, breathing deeply and slowly.

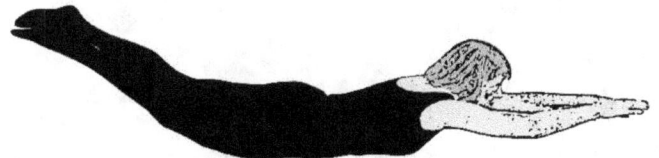

Return to the original resting position with your head turned to the side, and completely relax for 1 to 3 minutes.

## Stretch 8

This exercise helps relieve emotional tension and frustration. By helping release emotional upset locked in the muscles, this stretch promotes a sense of relaxation, mental balance, improved energy, and vitality.

Lie on your back with your hands interlaced under your neck. As you inhale, bend and lift your right leg.

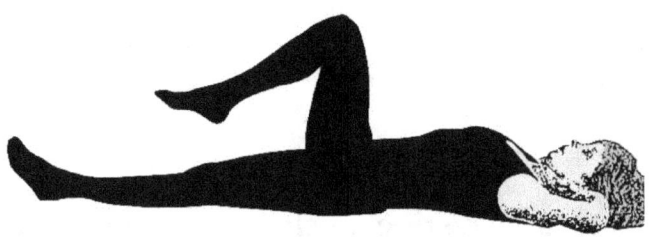

Then exhale and roll on your left side, with your left knee touching the ground. As you do this, release a sigh. As you inhale, return to your original position.

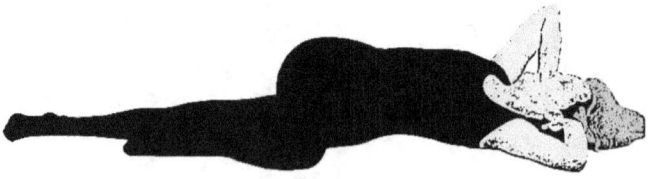

Repeat this 10 times, alternating sides. Then relax on your back for 1 minute.

*Stretch 9*

This exercise helps relieve PMS- and menopause-related anxiety and stress and other premenstrual and menopausal symptoms by energizing the female reproductive tract. It also energizes the liver, intestines, and kidneys, and strengthens the lower back, abdomen, buttocks, and legs.

Lie face down on the floor. Make fists with both your hands and place them under your hips. This prevents compression of the lumbar spine while doing the exercise.

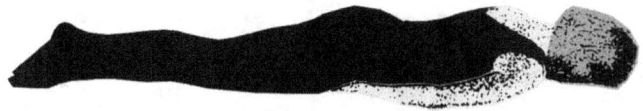

Straighten your body and raise your right leg with a slow upward thrust as high as you can, keeping your hips on your fists. Hold for 5 to 20 seconds if possible.

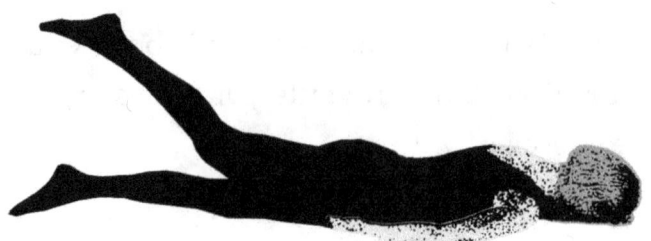

Lower the leg and slowly return to your original position. Repeat with the left leg, then with both legs together. Remember to keep your hips resting on your fists. Repeat 10 times.

*Stretch 10*

This exercise is one of the most powerful stretches for increasing total body energy and vitality and releasing muscle tension. It strengthens the nervous system, balances the mood, may reduce sugar craving, and helps reduce anxiety and nervous tension. It improves concentration and mental clarity. It also stimulates the thyroid, thymus, liver, kidneys, and female reproductive tract, and improves digestive function.

Lie face down on the floor, arms at your sides.

Slowly bend your legs at the knees and bring your feet up toward your buttocks.

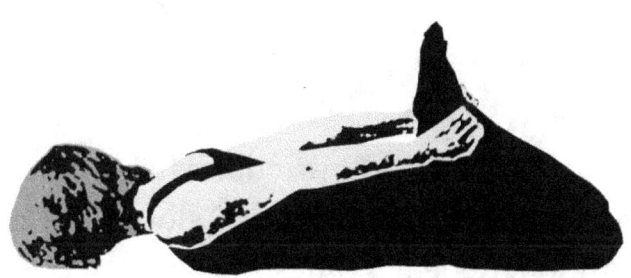

Reach back with your arms and carefully take hold of first one foot and then the other. Flex your feet to make grasping them easier.

Inhale and raise your trunk from the floor as far as possible. Lift your head and elevate your knees off the floor.

Squeeze the buttocks. Imagine your body looking like a gently curved bow. Hold for 10 to 15 seconds.

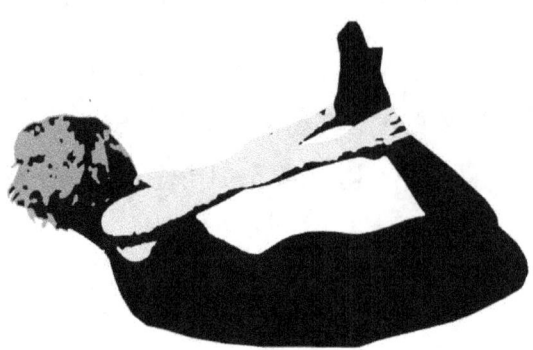

Slowly release the posture. Allow your chin to touch the floor and finally release your feet and return them slowly to the floor. Return to your original position. Repeat 5 times.

## Stretch 11

This exercise helps relieve nervous tension and stress, tension headaches, and menstrual problems. It also helps prevent colds and respiratory infections. Use it to relieve allergic and respiratory symptoms.

Lie on your back with your knees bent and the bottoms of your feet flat on the floor

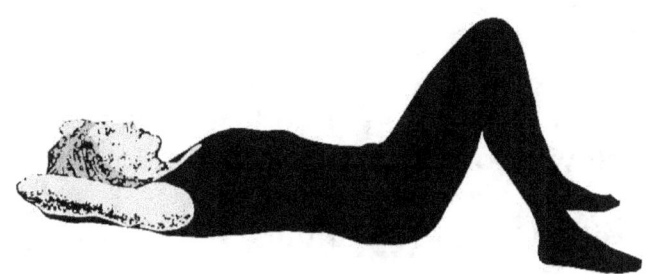

Bring your hands under your neck with the backs of your hands pressing against each other and the knuckles of your smallest fingers pressing into the base of your skull. Spread your index finger and thumb apart on each hand.

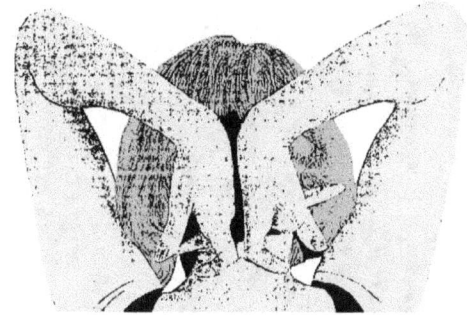

Inhale deeply and arch your hips up. Breathe deeply in this position for up to 1 minute.

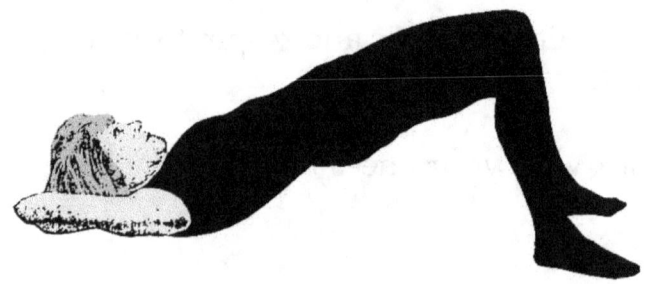

As you exhale, slowly come down and return to your original position.

Relax in this position for 1 to 3 minutes.

# 13

## Acupressure for Relief of Anxiety and Stress

Acupressure helps relieve both the emotional and the physical causes of anxiety and stress. Based on an ancient Chinese healing technique, it involves applying gentle finger pressure to specific points on the skin. Unlike acupuncture, which requires the use of needles and many years of training, acupressure can be easily learned and performed.

I have recommended the use of simple acupressure points to my patients for many years, and I have been pleased with the positive feedback they give me. Many of them have told me that they feel calmer and more peaceful after working with acupressure. This chapter includes easy-to-follow directions and many photographs of specific exercises, which should make acupressure easy for you.

### About Acupressure

Pressing specific acupressure points creates changes on two levels. On the physical level, acupressure affects muscular tension, blood circulation, and other physiological parameters. On a more subtle level, according to Traditional Chinese Medicine, acupressure also builds the body's life energy, thereby promoting healing. In fact, acupressure is based on the belief that the body contains a life energy called chi. It is different from, yet similar to, electromagnetic energy. Health can be viewed as a state in which the chi is equally distributed throughout the body and is present in sufficient amounts to energize all the cells and tissues of the body.

The chi energy runs through the body in channels called meridians. When working in a healthy manner, these channels distribute the energy evenly throughout the body, sometimes on the surface of the skin and at times deep inside the body in the organs. Disease occurs when the energy flow in a meridian is blocked or stopped. As a result, the internal organs that correspond to the meridians can show symptoms of disease. The meridian flow can be corrected by stimulating the points on the skin surface by hand massage. When the normal flow of energy through the body is resumed, the body is believed to heal itself spontaneously. Follow the simple instructions and stimulate the acupressure points using finger pressure. It is safe and painless, and does not require the use of needles.

## How to Perform Acupressure

Do the acupressure by yourself or with a friend when you are relaxed. Have your room warm and quiet. Make sure your hands are clean and nails trimmed (to avoid bruising yourself). If you tend to have cold hands, put them under warm water.

Work on the side of the body that has the most discomfort. If both sides are equally uncomfortable, choose whichever one you want. Working on one side seems to relieve the symptoms on both sides. Energy or information seems to transfer from one side to the other.

To find the correct acupressure point, look in the photograph accompanying the instructions. Each point corresponds to a specific point on the acupressure meridians. You may massage the points once a day or more during the time that you have symptoms.

Hold each indicated point with a steady pressure for one to three minutes. Apply pressure slowly with the tips or balls of the fingers. Make sure your hand is comfortable. Place several fingers over the area of the point. If you feel resistance or tension in the area to which you are applying pressure, you may want to push a little harder. However, if your hand starts to feel tense or tired, lighten the pressure a bit. The acupressure point may feel somewhat tender. This means the energy pathway or meridian is blocked.

During the treatment, the tenderness in the point should slowly go away. You may also have a subjective feeling of energy radiating from this point into the body. Many patients describe this sensation as very pleasant. Don't worry if you don't feel it—not everyone does. The main goal is relief from your symptoms. Breathe gently while doing each exercise. As you become more relaxed, your body will respond to the changes in the energy flow.

## *Exercise 1: Use for Relief of Anxiety and Stress*

This exercise helps relieve anxiety, nervous tension, and insomnia. It can also help relieve anxiety coexisting with mitral valve pro-lapse. It stimulates the entire endocrine system because it involves a powerful point for the pituitary gland. The points in this exercise also help relieve headaches, stiff neck, and stress-related breathing difficulties. This is also an effective exercise for relieving menopause-related hot flashes and hypoglycemia symptoms.

Sit upright on a chair. Hold each step for 1 to 3 minutes. Left hand holds spot located in the slight depression on the top of the head. Right hand holds point directly between the eyebrows where the bridge of the nose meets the forehead.

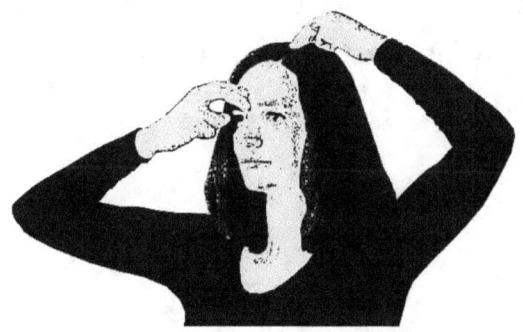

Right hand holds point in the center of your breastbone, at the level of the heart. Your fingers will fit into the indentations in this bone.

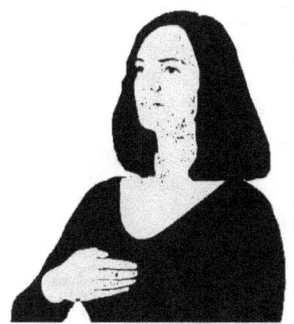

## Exercise 2: Use for Relief of Muscle Tension, Stress, and Hypoglycemia

Women who feel anxious and stressed often suffer from tight muscles. This important sequence of points helps relieve upper body tension. The neck and shoulders generally carry a great deal of tension. Tightness in this area can act as a bottleneck and impede the energy flow of the entire body. Thus, this sequence energizes the entire body, relieving fatigue and burnout as well as relieving anxiety and nervous tension. The points in this sequence strengthen the immune system and also include a major treatment point for hypoglycemia.

Hold each step 1 to 3 minutes. You will begin in a lying-down position and then sit upright on a chair.

Fold a towel in half lengthwise. Lie down on your back and place the towel underneath your upper back between your shoulder blades, applying pressure to an important pressure point. Relax in this position for 1 to 3 minutes.

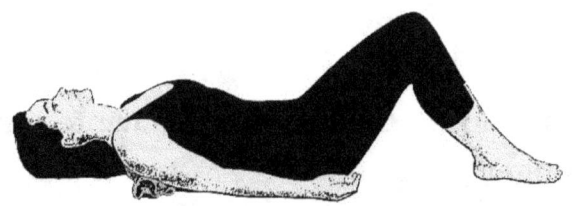

Now sit up. Left hand holds a point at the top of the shoulder blade, 1 to 2 inches to the side of the spine. The point is between the shoulder blade and the spine. It may feel firm and resistant.

Right hand holds the same point on the right side.

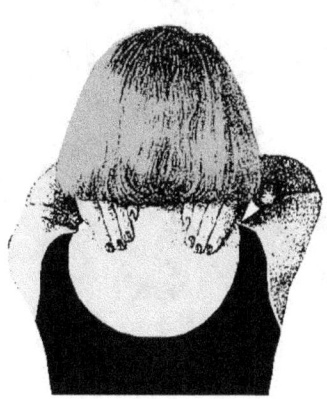

Left hand holds a point slightly to the back of the top of the shoulder where the neck meets the shoulder.

Right hand holds the same point on the right side.

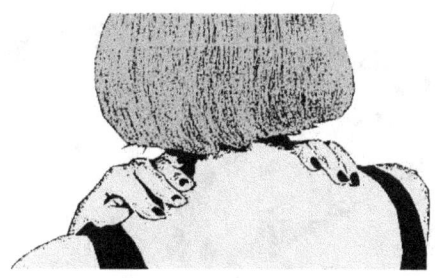

Left hand holds the point halfway on the neck; fingers rest on the muscle next to the spine.

Right hand holds the same point on the right side.

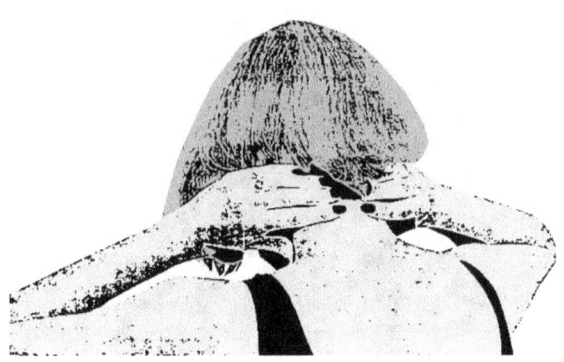

Left hand holds the point underneath the base of the skull, 1 to 2 inches out from the spine. Your fingers will feel a hollow spot at this point.

Right hand holds the point on the right side.

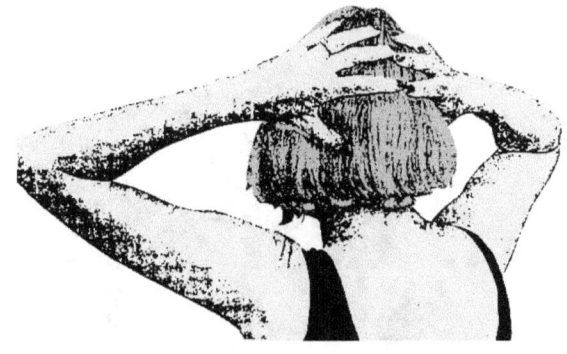

## Exercise 3: Use for Relief of Insomnia

This exercise helps relieve insomnia and anxiety. In Traditional Chinese Medicine, these points are called "joyful sleep" and "calm sleep."

Sit comfortably and hold these points for 1 to 3 minutes.

Left hand holds the point on the inside of the right ankle. This point is located in the indentation directly below the inner ankle bone.

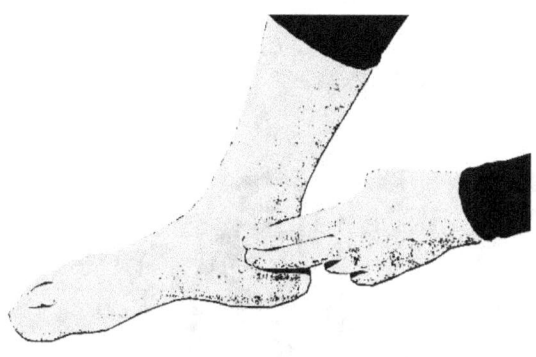

Right hand holds the point located in the indentation below the right outer ankle.

Repeat this exercise holding the points on the left foot.

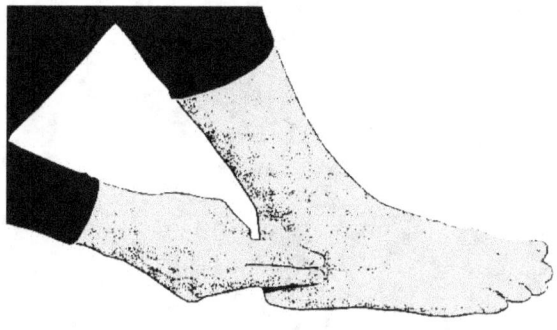

## *Exercise 4: Use to Relieve Chest Tension*

This exercise relieves chest tension and shallow breathing caused by anxiety. It also involves a point that reduces hypoglycemia symptoms.

Sit comfortably. Hold each point 1 to 3 minutes.

Left hand holds the point on the outer part of the chest. This point is located three finger widths below the collarbone.

Right hand holds the same point on the right side.

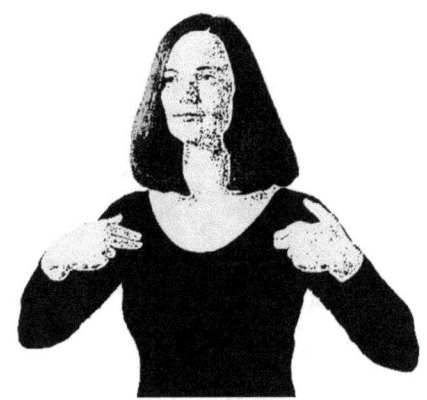

Left hand holds a point on the right hand below the base of the thumb, in the wrist groove.

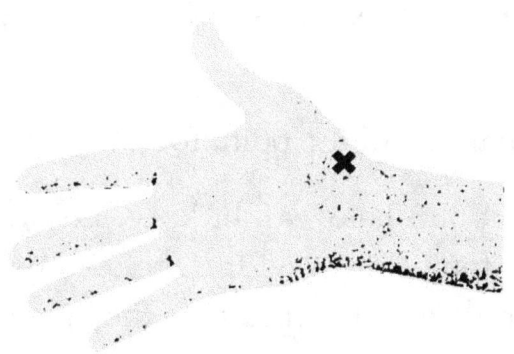

Left hand holds a point on the palm side of the right hand in the center of the pad below the thumb.

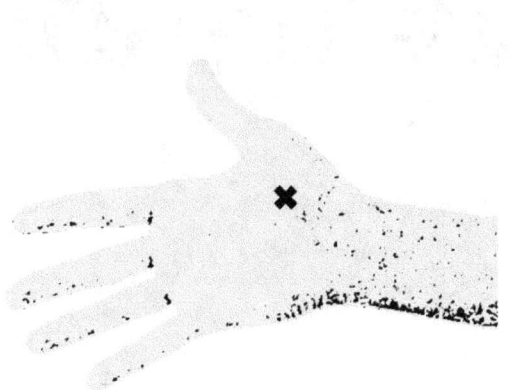

*Exercise 5: Use for Relief of Digestive Tension*

This powerful energy point is one of the most important in Traditional Chinese Medicine. It helps relieve digestive problems due to nervous tension and anxiety. It is also used to quickly diminish fatigue and improve energy and endurance. It has traditionally been used by athletes to tone and strengthen the muscles as well as increase stamina.

Sit upright on a chair. Hold the point for 1 to 3 minutes

Left hand holds a point below right knee. Locate this point with right hand, measuring four finger widths below the kneecap toward the outside of the shinbone. It is sensitive to the in many people.

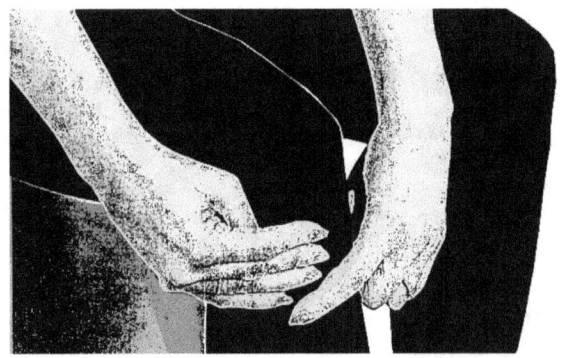

## *Exercise 6: Relieves PMS and Menstrual-Related Anxiety*

This exercise relieves PMS symptoms and menstrual cramps by balancing points on the bladder meridian. This meridian relieves symptoms by balancing the energy of the female reproductive tract. Traditional Chinese Medicine uses these points to relieve anxiety, fear, and exhaustion related to PMS, cramps, and other reproductive problems.

Sit on the floor and prop your back against a wall or a heavy piece of furniture. Hold each step for 1 to 3 minutes.

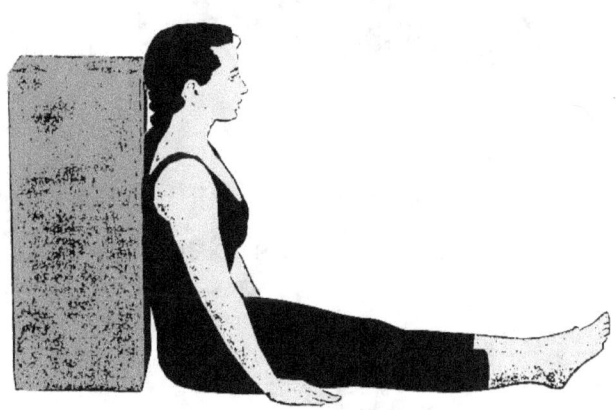

Alternative method: Lie on the floor and put your lower legs over the seat of a chair. Follow the exercise from that position.

Place left hand 1 inch above the waist on the muscle to the left side of the spine (muscle will feel firm and ropelike). Place right hand behind crease of the left knee.

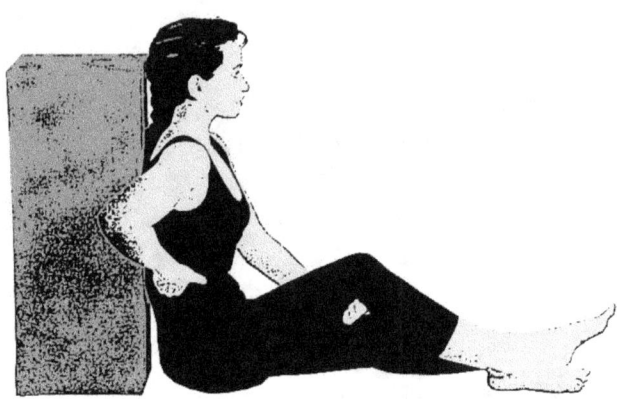

Left hand stays in the same position. Right hand is placed on the center of the back of the left calf. This is just below the fullest part of the calf.

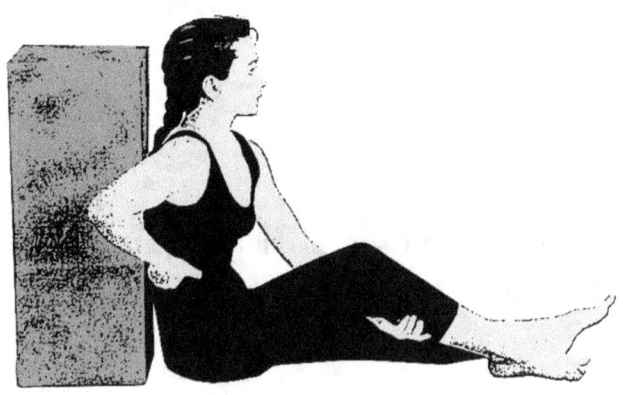

Left hand remains 1 inch above the waist on the muscle to the side of the spine. Right hand is placed just below the ankle bone on the outside of the left heel.

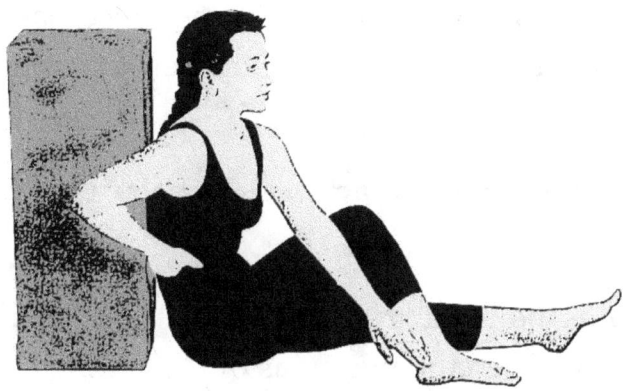

Left hand remains 1 inch above the waist on the muscle to the side of the spine. Right hand holds the front and back of the left little toe at the nail.

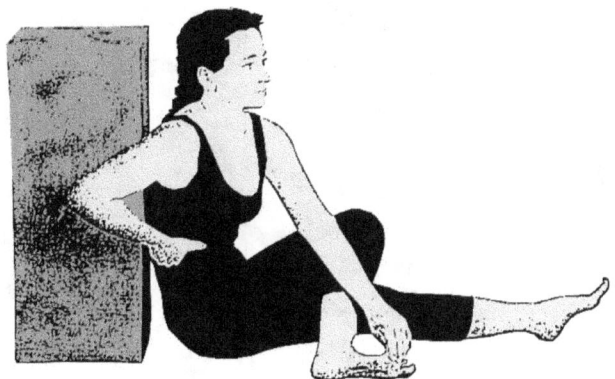

## Exercise 7: Relieves Menstrual Stress and Fatigue

This exercise helps relieve menstrual anxiety and depression, helpful to women suffering from significant stress in their lives. It helps relieve hot flashes related to the onset of menopause, as well as breathing difficulties caused by anxiety. The sequence of points relieves fatigue that many women experience for up to several days prior to the onset of their menstrual period. The second step in this sequence has traditionally been forbidden for use by pregnant women after their first trimester.

Sit up and prop your back against a chair. Hold each step 1 to 3 minutes.

Right hand holds point at the base of the ball of the right foot. This point is located between the two pads of the foot.

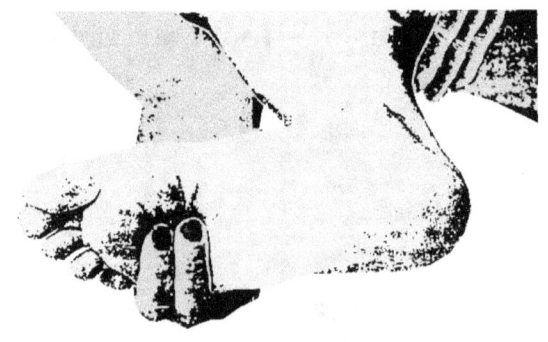

Left hand holds the point midway between the inside of the right anklebone and the Achilles tendon. The Achilles tendon is located at the back of the ankle.

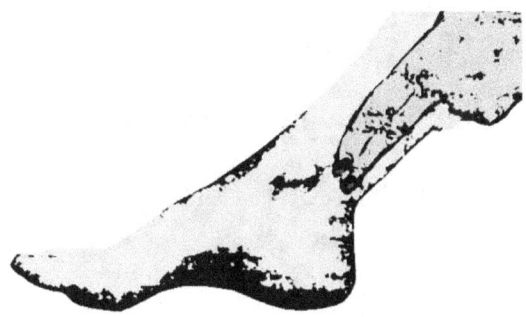

Left hand holds a point below right knee. Locate this point with right hand, measuring four finger widths below the kneecap toward the outside of the shinbone. It is sensitive to the in many people.

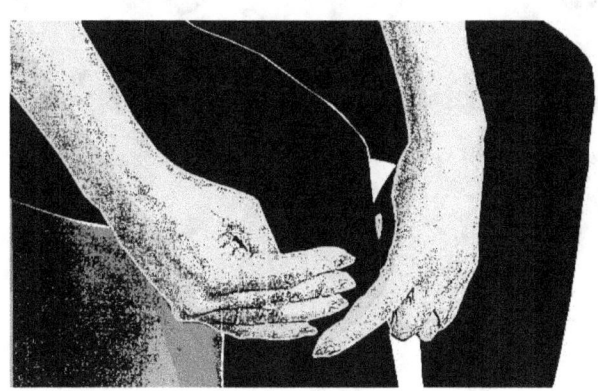

### *Exercise 8: Use to Balance the Thyroid Gland*

These points help balance the thyroid gland and normalize thyroid function. They also promote healthy skin tone and color.

Sit or lie in a comfortable position. Hold each step for 1 to 3 minutes.

Left hand holds a point in the indentation behind the ear lobe.

Left hand holds a point directly below the ear lobe and behind the jawbone.

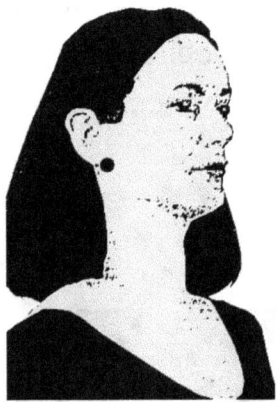 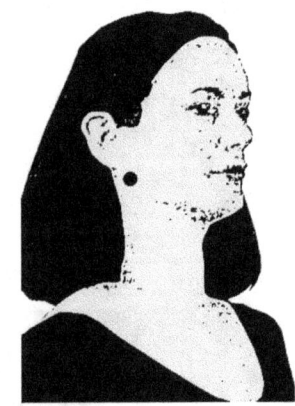

### *Exercise 9: Use to Balance the Thyroid Gland*

This exercise balances the thyroid gland. A hyperactive gland can cause anxiety and nervousness.

Sit upright on a chair. Hold each step for 1 to 3 minutes.

Wrap hands around shoulders with thumbs pressing gently into both sides on top of collarbone.

Fingers are in back. Press against upper shoulders and shoulder blade area.

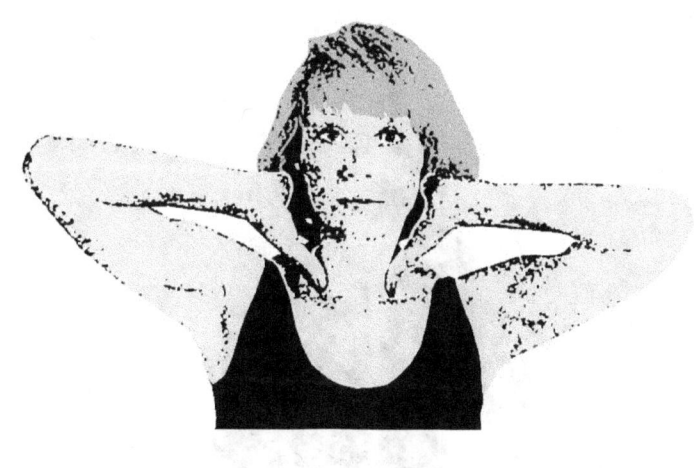

## Exercise 10: Use for Relief of Food Addiction

This exercise helps relieve food cravings and addictions for foods that worsen anxiety and nervous tension. This includes chocolate, sugar, and caffeine. This exercise also helps relieve anxiety and emotional stress, which often worsen digestive problems. Use this point on an empty stomach prior to eating. Do not hold this point deeply.

Sit or lie in a comfortable position. Hold this point for 1 to 3 minutes.

Right hand holds a point in the midline of the body, halfway between the bottom of the breast bone and the navel.

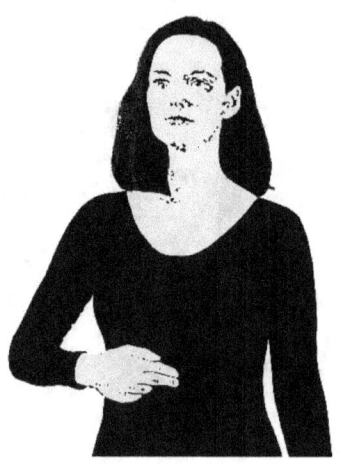

# 14

## Treating Anxiety, Panic Attacks and Phobias with Drugs

Though this book has emphasized the importance and effectiveness of self-care techniques for the treatment of anxiety and stress, medication also has a proper place in some circumstances. This is particularly true when symptoms of anxiety are severe and are affecting your ability to function effectively in your life.

If this is your situation, then you may want to consider going on medication while you are improving your ability to handle stress and bringing your brain chemistry into better balance through the self-care therapies discussed in this book. This will be equally true for you whether you suffer from emotionally-based causes of anxiety or have certain physical problems that cause anxiety, such as PMS, menopause, hyperthyroidism, and mitral valve prolapse.

However, it is important to remember that while medication can be very helpful, it shouldn't be thought of as a cure for your anxiety issues. While medication can provide temporary relief, it doesn't correct the underlying causes of your symptoms. Once you stop taking the medication, you may experience withdrawal symptoms and your anxiety symptoms will likely recur if you haven't treated the chemical and hormonal imbalances causing this condition. It is equally important to practice the effective self-care treatments and stress management techniques that I share with you in my book for a more calm, relaxed and joyful life.

Medication always needs to be prescribed by your physician or psychiatrist. If you decide to go on medication, it is important to work with a doctor that you trust and feel comfortable talking about your issues and concerns with. Good communication is important if you are the have the best response to a medication and avoid the pitfall and side effects that often go along with drug treatments.

I am going to describe some of the guidelines that I have followed with my own patients in approaching the use of medication for anxiety and panic attacks. You may find these guidelines helpful in dealing with your own situation.

## Drugs as Appropriate Therapy

In my own medical practice, I have tended to use drugs as a second line of treatment. I approach the use of drugs cautiously because of their powerful chemical effects on the body and potential for causing toxic side effects and addiction to the medication. My preference is to use the safer and gentler natural therapies such as diet, supplemental nutrients, stress-reduction techniques, deep breathing exercises, counseling, and physical exercises as my first line of treatment whenever possible. Whether you choose to use anti-anxiety medication or not, your best long-term results will come from practicing these self-care therapies since they will train you to handle stress in a much more healthful and beneficial manner.

### Situations When Drugs Are Appropriate

Sometimes the use of antianxiety medication may be an absolute necessity for the well-being of the patient. This is often the case when the symptoms are so severe that they do not respond completely to the natural therapies.

Examples include anxiety, phobias, and panic attacks of such frequency and severity that they will not allow a woman to function and carry out her necessary daily activities, whether performing a job or taking care of children. Similarly, if a woman has such intense anxiety that it is difficult for her to be in social situations with friends, family or even dating situations. If a woman is single and wants a relationship, medication may be a useful step towards better functioning. Also, if the anxiety condition is causing too much emotional pain and distress, then medication is indicated, at least on a short-term basis.

Sometimes the symptoms of anxiety are secondary to a health issue, as discussed earlier in this book. In this case, medication may be an appropriate therapy. For example, women with severe menopause-related anxiety, mood swings, and associated symptoms, such as hot flashes or night sweats caused by hormonal deficiency, may require bioidentical hormonal replacement therapy. This may be necessary to give her the relief she needs and get her back to a level of emotional and physiological comfort. Similarly, I have seen patients with severe PMS related anxiety and mood swings have great relief of their symptoms with bioidentical progesterone therapy.

Often, to obtain the best results in treating anxiety and stress of all types, I combine the medication with natural therapies. This gives a woman the full range of available treatment options. It also emphasizes prevention as well as immediate symptom relief.

## Using Drugs Safely and Effectively

When using drugs for the treatment of anxiety, I always try to prescribe medication only for short-term use and at the lowest therapeutic dose. Unfortunately, drug addiction and unpleasant side effects are real possibilities with the long-term use of many anxiety reducing drugs, particularly at high doses. The judicious and careful use of these medications reduces the risk of unpleasant side effects, as well as the withdrawal symptoms that can occur when drugs are discontinued.

Before embarking on a medication program, make sure you understand both the risks and benefits of the medications that you are considering. Discuss the potential side effects and any contraindications to normal activities with your physician when using these drugs.

For example, if a drug causes sedative effects, you should not attempt to drive a car when these side effects are pronounced. Find out how long your physician plans to keep you on medication and after what time period it will be discontinued to avoid withdrawal effects. Your physician should have a good plan in mind when beginning a program that includes medication.

## Good Communication with Your Doctor is Essential

I have always been aware of how important good communication is with my own patients in order to create the best treatment results. I always strive to provide an environment in which my patients feel safe and comfortable in discussing any concerns or issues with me.

It is important that my patients feel that they can ask me any questions or discuss any concerns that they might have. To support this process, I have always set aside plenty of time to talk with my patients during their sessions so that they don't feel that I am rushing to get to the next patient. I want my patients to feel that we are working together as a team and that they can count on me as a strong support system in their lives. This is the kind of medical care that I would want if I were a patient!

Medication always needs to be prescribed by your physician or psychiatrist. If you decide to go on medication, it is important to work with a doctor that you trust and feel comfortable talking about your issues and concerns with. Good communication is important if you are to have the best response to a medication and avoid the pitfall and side effects that often go along with drug treatments.

To ensure that you have a positive experience with your own physician or caregiver, it is important to share certain information with him or her. For example, before you start on antianxiety medication, provide any information to your physician that could affect the use of a particular drug. Pertinent information includes data about any allergies or unusual reactions that you might have to drugs or any other substances, such as foods, preservatives, or dyes. You might also need to use medication for a particular health condition. For example, if you have mitral valve prolapse, you will need to use antibiotics prophylactically before dental work or surgery.

Be sure to notify your physician if you are currently taking any other prescription or over-the-counter medications. This will help prevent potentially dangerous drug interactions. Inform your physician if you are pregnant or breastfeeding, because the use of medications can be dangerous to the fetus or nursing infant. If you develop any new medical problem while you are using any of the prescription drugs that I discuss in this chapter, inform your physician immediately.

If you find communication with your physician difficult or you feel uncomfortable talking about your concerns, I suggest that you find another physician with whom you do feel comfortable. The decision about whether to use a particular medication requires a mutual decision on the part of the patient and physician, exchanging full information about the patient's condition and the risks and benefits of the drug. Such matters can be best discussed in a positive patient-doctor relationship.

In the following section of this chapter, I discuss the drugs used most commonly for both the emotional and physical causes of anxiety and stress. This should provide you with useful information when making a decision with your physician about drug therapy.

## Prescription Drugs

Four major types of prescription drugs can be useful in relieving anxiety, stress, and panic symptoms; benzodiazepine tranquilizers and sedatives, antidepressants, beta-blockers, and the anti-anxiety drug BuSpar (buspirone hydrochloride). I will share with you their uses and benefits as well as their potential side effects.

### Benzodiazepine Tranquilizers and Sedatives

Benzodiazepines are among the most commonly used medications for treating anxiety. They decrease anxiety by slowing down the central nervous system and reducing brain activity. They have relaxing and calming effects which many patients find helpful. These medications have sedative properties, too, depending on the dosage.

Some women find them helpful in promoting better sleep if they are suffering from anxiety related insomnia. Benzodiazepines tend to be fast acting. They usually provide symptom relief within 30 minutes to one hour which can be very helpful if you are suffering from a panic attack or severe anxiety episode that you are finding difficult to manage.

Pharmaceutical companies have developed and isolated more than two thousand benzodiazepine formulas and tested over one hundred of them for anti-anxiety properties. Benzodiazepines are divided into two groups: tranquilizers and sedatives.

Of the first group, benzodiazepine tranquilizers, Xanax (alprazolam), Ativan (lorezepam), Valium (diazepam), Tranxene (clorazepate), and Klonopin (clonazepam) are most commonly prscribed for acute anxiety on a short-term basis. In lower doses they can be used for panic disorders on a longer-term basis. Anafranil (clomipramine) is used as an alternative therapy for patients suffering from obsessive disorder who do not respond well to antidepressants (discussed later on in this section.) Physicians and psychiatrists also prescribe these drugs to treat women with PMS- and menopause-related anxiety as well as women with eating disorders, especially food addiction coexisting with anxiety.

In high doses, the tranquilizers behave like sedatives; thus, they can also be used to induce sleep. Certain tranquilizers like Valium reduce muscle tension and spasm, which is sometimes aggravated in women who suffer from excessive anxiety and stress. Other tranquilizers like Librium may be combined with a second antispasmodic drug to create drugs like Librax, which reduces both anxiety and smooth muscle spasm. Conditions like irritable bowel syndrome, commonly triggered by anxiety and stress, respond well to these combinations.

Several of the tranquilizers are also used to treat the anxiety associated with alcohol withdrawal; these include Librium, which is beneficial because of its anticonvulsant effects, and Valium because it provides safety against alcohol overdose. These two drugs can be given intravenously to alcoholics, a benefit for people who react to the oral drugs with nausea and vomiting. Short-acting benzodiazepines like Serax (oxazepam) are used less frequently for alcohol withdrawal.

The second group, benzodiazepine sedatives ("sleeping pills"), includes Dalmane (flurazepam), Halcion (triazolam), Restoril (temazepam), and AtivanBenzodia (lorazepam). These sedatives are very effective in inducing a state of deep and refreshing sleep when first started. They are useful on a short-term basis and for women with severe acute anxiety as well as insomnia caused by menopause and PMS episodes. With continuing use, however, the patient develops a tolerance to the drugs and the doses need to be gradually increased. This brings with it the risk of increased side effects as well as withdrawal symptoms when therapy is discontinued. Thus, these drugs should preferably be used only for short courses of therapy.

Because all the benzodiazepines have similar mechanisms of action, they differ mainly in how long they stay in your body (called their "half-life") after the liver breaks down the components into chemical metabolites. The metabolites are the form in which they're excreted from your body. Some benzodiazepines like Valium and Dalmane have long half-lives, while Xanax and Halcion tend to have short half-lives and are excreted rapidly.

Benzodiazepine tranquilizers and sedatives have similar side effects including drowsiness, lethargy, fatigue, and "morning hangover." Other side-effects include confusion and disorientation, slurred speech, dizziness, impaired thinking, memory loss and even depression. Occasionally, paradoxic reactions can occur within the first few weeks of therapy. These reactions are characterized by an increase in anxiety, irritability, rage, insomnia, and even hallucinations.

When benzodiazepine tranquilizers and sedatives are prescribed for long periods of time (more than several months), withdrawal symptoms may occur on discontinuing therapy. This is because the long-term use of these drugs can result in physical and psychological addiction. Tolerance can develop and the dosages have to be increased over time to continue to get a therapeutic effect. Abrupt withdrawal can produce symptoms similar to alcohol withdrawal. Milder withdrawal symptoms include insomnia, weakness, and anxiety. More severe symptoms include seizures and delirium. Ideally, withdrawal of benzodiazepines should take place gradually over a two- to four-week period.

In summary, the benzodiazepine medications have a wide range of uses for the treatment of anxiety, irritability, insomnia, and muscle tension caused by both emotional and physical problems, including acute anxiety, panic disorders, PMS, menopause, food addiction, and alcohol abuse.

However, because of side effects and drug tolerances that increase with elevations in the dose, and because of the problem of drug dependency that can develop over time, these drugs should be prescribed only for short periods of time. Also, they are not curative. Eighty percent of women report recurrence of their anxiety symptoms once the drugs are stopped. Thus, while these medications can relieve symptoms temporarily, a combination of natural self-help therapies and counseling is needed to prevent a recurrence of anxiety symptoms on a long-term basis.

## Antidepressants

Antidepressants are the medications most commonly used to treat depression if it coexists with anxiety. They are also used to treat panic attacks or agoraphobia with panic attacks. Antidepressants are also often prescribed for women with PMS and menopause who suffer from mood symptoms.

The most commonly prescribed drugs today for the treatment of anxiety as well as depression are the selective serotonin reuptake inhibitors (SSRIs). These medications are also helpful for obsessive-compulsive disorder and post-traumatic stress disorder. These medications work by blocking a receptor in the brain that reabsorbs serotonin. This helps to change the balance of serotonin, thereby supporting brain cells to send and receive chemical messages. The end result is an improvement in mood and behavior is women with PMS related depression and depression in general. Commonly prescribed SSRI's include Prozac (fluoxetine), Celexa (citalopram), Zoloft (sertraline) and Paxil (paroxetine).

The main drawback with these medications is that they are slow to be effective. To begin to feel symptom relief may take between two to eight weeks, so you may not feel better when you initially begin to take these medications. It is important, however, to keep taking them since they are likely to be beneficial once their therapeutic effects start to manifest.

Unlike other mood altering drugs, SSRIs antidepressants are not physically addictive, so the threat of developing withdrawal symptoms is not an issue. However, some women become psychologically addicted to the antidepressants and may have a difficult time weaning themselves off medication. Other side effects include nausea, dry mouth, nervousness, agitation, headache, diarrhea, reduced sexual desire, insomnia and weight gain.

Women who have been taking these medications for a period of time may find that they develop withdrawal symptoms if these medications are abruptly discontinued. They should be gradually tapered off so that the brain can readjust to lower levels of these drugs.

Once the antidepressants are stopped, the symptoms may recur, but less frequently than is experienced by women taking benzodiazepines. Recurrence rate runs between 25 and 50 percent (contrasted with approximately 80 to 90 percent for benzodiazepines). The use of these medications for at least six months may also help prevent the recurrence of depression for a longer period of time.

Tricyclic antidepressants, commonly known as "mood elevators," are an older class of antidepressants that are still commonly used today. They produce both an antidepressant and mild tranquilizing effect. Because it takes some time to build up to a therapeutic effect once treatment is initiated, there is a dangerous period of time before the drug takes hold when the patient may remain depressed and become suicidal. However, after two to three weeks of treatment, 80 percent of depressed and anxious patients notice an elevation of mood, increased alertness, and improvement in appetite.

Common tricyclic medications include Elavil (amitriptyline), Tofranil (imipramine), Aventyl (nortriptyline), Norpramin (desipramine) and Sinequan (doxepin). While the actual mechanism of action is not known, it is thought that depression is relieved by elevating the neurotransmitters levels like serotonin and norepinephrine. These are chemicals present in the brain that regulate mood, personality, sleep, and appetite. Many women with depression may lack adequate levels of these neurotransmitters.

Which of these antidepressants are best suited for panic episodes, agoraphobia, and anxiety coexisting with depression varies from person to person. The efficiency of any antidepressant depends on each individual's body chemistry. As a result, the patient may have to try several antidepressants to find the one that produces the best therapeutic effect.

Side effects of these drugs are fairly common. In fact, as many as one-quarter of all patients stop therapy with these drugs because of the unpleasant side effects. Many women using antidepressants will initially complain of dry mouth, blurred vision, constipation, drowsiness, weight gain, fatigue, headaches, nausea and even rarely seizures. These symptoms tend to fade in intensity after the first few weeks of taking the medication.

In summary, tricyclic antidepressants can produce much benefit in the short- to intermediate-term treatment of anxiety coexisting with depression, panic episodes, and agoraphobia. They're also useful for the treatment of PMS- and menopause-related depression. However, side effects are common and psychological dependency can develop.

### Antianxiety

BuSpar (buspirone hydrochloride) is a very useful anti-anxiety drug that has two definite benefits over benzodiazepines and other sedatives. First, it does not cause excessive levels of sedation, so the potentially debilitating side effect of drowsiness is decreased. Second, it is not addictive, so women using BuSpar do not run the risk of becoming dependent on this drug or having to go through a potentially uncomfortable withdrawal period in order to discontinue it. As a result, some physicians favor it over traditional drugs such as Xanax for regular use in treating generalized anxiety. Women suffering from fear, worry, tension, and irritability may benefit from this medication. It is also useful for treating the anxiety component when anxiety and depression coexist. It is less useful, however, in treating panic attacks.

Though BuSpar is a relatively safe drug; it should not be used with antidepressant medication belonging to the monoamine oxidase inhibitor (MAO inhibitor) classification. Interaction of these two drugs may cause an elevation in blood pressure. Also, even though BuSpar has been found to be less sedating than other anti-anxiety drugs, a woman taking it should avoid operating an automobile until she is sure that the drug does not affect her mental and motor performance.

Nervous system side effects such as drowsiness, dizziness, nervousness, and insomnia of sufficient severity to necessitate discontinuing use of the drug were seen in 3.4 percent of 2200 women studied in a clinical trial. This trial was done during the preapproval stage of testing to gather the necessary data so that the drug could be sold in the United States. In the same clinical trial, 1.2 percent of the women tested experienced digestive disturbances such as nausea severe enough to necessitate discontinuing the drug. Other reported side effects include chest pain, tinnitus (ringing in the ears), dream disturbances, sore throat, and nasal congestion.

The good news is that the side effects occur in a relatively small number of patients using the drug, however. For women who tolerate the drug well, the lack of physical dependence or potential for drug abuse make it a drug of choice for the treatment of generalized anxiety beta blockers.

These drugs are primarily used to treat conditions triggered by hyperactivity of the sympathetic nervous system. This is the part of the nervous system that triggers the fight-or-flight response, with increased heart and pulse rate. Beta blockers such as Inderal™ (propranolol hydrochloride) help reduce nervous system hyperactivity by blocking the transmission of nerve impulses to the beta receptors of the sympathetic nervous system. These receptors are found in abundance in the nerves that control the heart muscle. By slowing down the heart rate, these drugs relieve such stress-sensitive problems as cardiac arrhythmia (irregular or overly fast heartbeat), high blood pressure, and migraine headaches.

Inderal is also commonly used to treat anxiety, particularly when accompanied by physical symptoms such as heart palpitations or rapid heartbeat. It is particularly useful when taken as a single dose to relieve anxiety symptoms that may precede a stressful situation like public speaking, examinations or a job interview. Women with mitral valve prolapse are more prone to panic attacks than the general population, for reasons that are not yet understood. In women with this condition, the use of Inderal can help to control rapid or irregular heartbeat and anxiety episodes.

The use of Inderal should be avoided altogether or monitored carefully in women with pre-existing congestive heart failure or asthma, because the use of this drug may worsen these conditions. Inderal may help relieve the symptoms of hyperthyroidism, a physical cause of anxiety. However, it should be used carefully because it may mask clinical signs of conditions such as tachycardia, making it difficult to evaluate the severity of underlying conditions. While slowing the heart rate is beneficial for women with hyperthyroidism, discontinuing the Inderal may worsen the symptoms and put the patient at risk of precipitating a thyroid crisis.

Women with anxiety symptoms who do not have these potentially dangerous preexisting conditions may use Inderal with reasonable safety. Common side effects include excessive slowing of the heart rate, lowering of blood pressure, lightheadedness, fatigue, weakness, drowsiness, nausea, vomiting, and abdominal cramping. If Inderal is prescribed on a regular basis, withdrawal symptoms can occur, so use of the drug should be stopped gradually over a sufficient period of time.

## Drugs for PMS

Several drug therapies are available for the treatment of PMS-related anxiety, mood swings, and increased sensitivity to stress. These include progesterone as well as mood-altering drugs like the benzodiazepine tranquilizers and antidepressants. I discuss the use of progesterone here. For information on tranquilizers and antidepressants, see the preceding discussion.

## Progesterone

Progesterone is a hormone secreted by the ovaries after ovulation, present along with estrogen during the second half of the menstrual cycle. Since PMS also begins after ovulation, many suspect that imbalances in the levels of estrogen and progesterone cause PMS, particularly the emotional symptoms. (80 to 90 percent of women with PMS complain of anxiety and mood swings from several days to two weeks each month.) Since both estrogen and progesterone affect brain chemistry as well as mood, this is a particularly interesting hypothesis. Excessive levels of estrogen are linked to anxiety and irritability, while progesterone has a sedative effect on the brain.

This was corroborated in an early research study that was reported in the *Journal of Assisted Reproduction and Genetics*. This study found that the use of 200 mg of progesterone vaginal suppositories used twice daily for 7 months effectively reduced PMS-related symptoms

Progesterone also increases the brain's output of its own opiates, such as beta-endorphins, which help promote a sense of emotional well-being. When the balance between the two female hormones is tipped in favor of one hormone or the other, emotional symptoms can occur. This certainly occurs in younger women on the birth control pill or in menopausal women on hormonal replacement therapy. Symptoms of anxiety and edginess or depression and fatigue can occur if the hormonal mix provided by the pill is poorly matched to the patient's body type. Different dosages or formulas may have to be tried until the mix is right for a particular patient.

Unfortunately, the research studies that have been done on this issue show contradictory data. However, the medical research findings do not negate the positive experiences of many women with PMS who have used progesterone therapy. I have seen this with my own patients who have been thrilled with the benefits that they have enjoyed with progesterone therapy.

In fact, many women suffering from PMS feel that progesterone is the only medical treatment that finally helped to eradicate their anxiety. Often their physicians have prescribed a whole range of mood-altering drugs in order to relieve the more severe anxiety and mood swing symptoms without positive results. When they then try progesterone, many women obtain the symptom relief that they are looking for.

In my own practice, I prefer to use progesterone in women who have more severe PMS symptoms to accompany the natural therapies like diet, nutritional supplements, and stress management. My own impression has been that progesterone definitely helps to reduce PMS symptoms in women who can benefit from this therapy.

If you think that progesterone is the right therapy for you and your physician or caregiver does not see any health issues that might interfere with your use of this therapy, you may want to consider using bioidentical progesterone. Bioidentical progesterone is identical to the progesterone made by our own bodies. Progesterone is most commonly available as a skin cream or as a tablet to be taken orally. Progesterone skin cream can be bought in health food stores or through the Internet while the tablets, called Prometrium, need to be prescribed by your physician. It can also be used as rectal or vaginal suppositories, transdermal sprays and sublingual drops.

A range of progesterone creams, available without a prescription, contain anywhere from less than 2 mg to more than 400 mg of the hormone per jar. Pro-Gest cream, which contains more than 400 mg in a container, is one of the better-known brands. The cream is applied to the skin and absorbed into the general circulation and reaches more body tissues than oral progesterone, which is first metabolized by the liver and converted into three different compounds. A typical dosage of natural progesterone is 40 mg a day.

Start progesterone therapy three days before the onset of PMS symptoms. For example, if PMS symptoms normally begin five days before your menstrual period, you should start taking progesterone eight days before the expected onset of your period.

Side effects of progesterone therapy are quite rare. When natural progesterone is taken in normally prescribed amounts, there are no known side effects. However, very high doses can cause drowsiness, due to its sedative effect on the brain. If you use progesterone as a rectal or vaginal suppository, rarely, you can experience local irritation of the rectal or vulvar mucosa caused by the medium in which the progesterone is mixed, leakage of the progesterone from the vagina, and a slight increase in the incidence of yeast vaginitis. In women with irregular menstrual cycles, high doses of progesterone may delay the onset of menstruation.

This can be remedied by simply stopping the progesterone; menstrual bleeding will follow soon after.

## Drugs for Menopause

Estrogen and progesterone therapy is usually the drug treatment of choice for menopause-related anxiety and edginess. However, the use of tranquilizers and antidepressants may occasionally be necessary to help a woman through the more unstable phases of menopause. This is particularly true during the early stages of menopause when the hormonal swings can be erratic and abrupt.

Menopausal women who are under stress are particularly susceptible to wide mood swings as their hormonal levels drop from the higher levels of the active reproductive years to the lower levels typical of the postmenopausal period. These women may need both hormones and mood stabilizing drugs.

I discuss the use of estrogen and progesterone therapy here. For more information on the benefits and side effects of benzodiazepine tranquilizers and sedatives as well as antidepressants, please refer to the earlier section of this chapter.

## Hormonal Replacement Therapy

The issue of whether to use hormones or not is a question that most menopausal women pursue with their own physician as well as with friends and through reading materials. Statistically, estrogen and progestin use is much lower than most women suspect. Only 15 percent of women in the menopause and postmenopause age group actually use hormonal replacement therapy (HRT). The women who choose not to use HRT often do so because their symptoms are mild or absent or they have many concerns about the possible immediate and long-term side effects that could occur with the use of hormones.

This has become a major issue for women in menopause since 2002 after a government commissioned study, the Women's Health Initiative, found that HRT could increase the risk of breast cancer, heart attack, strokes and blood clots. Synthetic forms of progesterone, called progestins like Provera, have traditionally been prescribed for menopausal women.

Unfortunately, progestins can worsen fatigue and depression in susceptible women. Women with coexisting anxiety and depression should use them cautiously while conventional forms of estrogen therapy can sometimes worsen anxiety. While these negative findings have continued to accumulate in studies done since this time, other research trials have found that HRT does have benefits such as the reduction of vaginal pain, dryness and hot flashes.

For women with moderate to severe anxiety, irritability, depression, fatigue, and insomnia related to menopausal hormonal changes, the use of HRT can be very beneficial, when taken as bioidentical estrogen and progesterone therapy rather than conventional HRT. Many menopausal women find that hormonal replacement therapy helps their moods and gives their energy level a tremendous boost.

As mentioned in the section on PMS, bioidentical hormones are just like the hormones made by your own body while the conventional types of hormones commonly prescribed by physicians differ in their chemical makeup and how they affect your body. They are not, however, found in this form in nature but are synthesized from a plant chemical extracted from soy or yams and then converted in the laboratory to the actual hormone, such as estrogen.

Many of my patients have reported not only relief from hot flashes and vaginal dryness, but also reduction in anxiety and improved sex drive with the use of bioidentical hormones. Depression, the blues, and fatigue are often eradicated, as are insomnia and irritability.

Bioidentical estrogen is usually prescribed as a much lower potency form of estrogen, called estriol. Unlike the more powerful forms of estrogen, called estradiol and estrone, this weaker form of estrogen is much less likely to cause side effects while still delivering very beneficial therapeutic effects. Estriol can also be combined with small amounts of the other, more powerful, forms of this hormone.

Both bioidentical estrogen and progesterone can be taken orally, sublingually (held in the cheek or under the tongue), used topically as a skin cream, suppositories, or by injection. Estrogen can also be delivered as a patch while progesterone is not yet available in this form.

Many of my patients have reported not only relief from hot flashes and vaginal dryness, but also reduction in anxiety and improved sex drive with the use of bioidentical hormones. Depression, the blues, and fatigue are often eradicated, as are insomnia and irritability. Because they were using a lower potency, weaker form of estrogen and progesterone that is identical in molecular structure to the hormone made within the body, they also had less problems with uncomfortable side-effects. As a result, they tolerated the therapy better and were less likely to stop or abandon the treatment.

Because of the possible side effects of using conventional hormones, most physicians prescribe the lowest dose of both estrogen and progesterone that relieves symptoms. Much higher doses were used several decades ago, both in estrogen replacement therapy and in birth control pills, but the current trend is definitely toward smaller doses of hormones to achieve the same beneficial effects.

## Drugs for Hyperthyroidism

Excessive secretion of thyroid hormone may cause symptoms of anxiety and nervousness. While these symptoms are usually accompanied by physical symptoms such as sweating, weight loss, loose bowel movements, and rapid heartbeat, initially distinguishing between emotional causes of anxiety and hyperthyroidism in a particular patient may be difficult.

Once the diagnosis has been determined by thyroid function testing, the focus of treatment will be on halting the thyroid's excessive secretion of hormone. Suppressing the thyroid either surgically or through drugs is the treatment. Drug therapy for the suppression of the thyroid gland is discussed here as well as the use of beta blockers to treat the symptoms.

### *Propylthiouracil*

Propylthiouracil is an antithyroid drug that blocks the production of thyroid hormone within the gland itself. Propylthiouracil does not destroy hormone that has already been produced. As a result, it can take up to four to six weeks for elevated levels of thyroid hormone to return to normal. Once the thyroid level is within the normal range, the patient can be placed on a lower maintenance dose of the drug to keep the thyroid levels from rising again.

However, thyroid function tests must be monitored periodically to make sure that the levels don't fall too low, producing hypothyroidism. Alternatively, some physicians prefer to use propylthiouracil at higher doses until the patient's thyroid hormone drops to levels below the normal range. At this point, thyroid replacement therapy is instituted to bring the patient's thyroid levels back to normal.

Propylthiouracil is the treatment of choice in young women and children because it allows reproductive options to remain intact. It provides an alternative to surgical removal of the thyroid gland and avoids the risks and potential postoperative complications of surgery.

Other than hypothyroidism, which can be minimized with careful monitoring, side effects include a skin rash, which develops in 5 percent of patients. Other, less frequent side effects include headaches, muscle and joint aches, enlargements of lymph glands in the neck, and loss of the sense of taste.

The long-term use of the drug seems to help prevent recurrence of hyperthyroidism. In patients treated between eighteen and twenty-four months with propylthiouracil, between 50 and 70 percent had no recurrence of the disease after the drug dosage is slowly decreased and finally discontinued. Women having a recurrence after drug cessation may need further treatment with propylthiouracil, radioactive iodine, or surgery.

### Radioactive Iodine

In some cases, a radioactive isotope of iodine is administered simply by having the patient drink water treated with radioactive iodine. Colorless and tasteless, the water treated with radiation is quite dangerous to the thyroid gland. The radioactive iodine is selectively absorbed into the thyroid gland in high concentrations. It then acts to destroy the thyroid gland while posing no damage to other tissues in the body. As a result, excessive thyroid hormone levels fall. The hormones often slowly fall to the hypothyroid level within a few years of treatment. Since the hormone-producing cells of the thyroid are essentially destroyed, thyroid replacement therapy becomes necessary.

Therapy with radioactive iodine is generally used in women over 30 who have no further wish to bear children. This is because the radiation may be a possible cause of genetic damage. There is also an increased risk of the development of cancer with the use of this drug. Like propylthiouracil, it does offer a nonsurgical approach to the treatment of hyperthyroidism. Even with its potential side effects and permanent destruction of the thyroid gland itself, this alternative to surgery can prevent much debilitating wear and tear on the patient.

### Beta Blockers

As mentioned earlier in this chapter, beta blockers are primarily used to treat conditions triggered by hyperactivity of the sympathetic nervous system. This is the part of the nervous system that triggers the fight-or-flight response, with increased heart and pulse rate. Beta blockers such as Inderal™ (propranolol hydrochloride) help reduce nervous system hyperactivity by blocking the transmission of nerve impulses to the beta-type receptors of the sympathetic nervous system. These receptors are found in abundance in the nerves that control the heart muscle and slowing down the heart rate.

Inderal may help relieve the symptoms of hyperthyroidism, a physical cause of anxiety. However, it should be used carefully because it may mask clinical signs of conditions such as tachycardia, making it difficult to evaluate the severity of underlying conditions. While slowing the heart rate is beneficial for women with hyperthyroidism, discontinuing the Inderal may worsen the symptoms and put the patient at risk of precipitating a thyroid crisis.

Women with mitral valve prolapse are more prone to panic attacks than the general population, for reasons that are not yet understood. In women with this condition, the use of Inderal can help to control rapid or irregular heartbeat and anxiety episodes.

The use of Inderal should be avoided altogether or monitored carefully in women with pre-existing congestive heart failure or asthma, because the use of this drug may worsen these conditions. Common side effects include excessive slowing of the heart rate, lowering of blood pressure, light-headedness, fatigue, weakness, drowsiness, nausea, vomiting, and abdominal cramping. If Inderal is prescribed on a regular basis, withdrawal symptoms can occur, so drug use should be stopped gradually over a sufficient period of time.

In summary, a wide variety of drugs offer the possibility of real symptom relief for emotional and physical causes of severe anxiety. All drugs run the risk of causing both short-term and long-term side effects, however. Before beginning any drug therapy, a woman should discuss possible risks and benefits with her physician. This allows for the best possible choice of medication, and the smallest chance of adverse side effects.

## Prescription Drugs

### Anxiety and depression

- Benzodiazepine tranquilizers
- Benzodiazepine sedatives
- Antidepressants
- Beta-blockers
- Antianxiety

### Food addiction

- Antidepressants

### PMS

- Progesterone
- Benzodiazepine tranquilizers
- Antidepressants

### Menopause

- Estrogen and progesterone (either natural or synthetic)
- Benzodiazepine tranquilizers
- Benzodiazepine sedatives
- Antidepressants

### Hyperthyroidism

- Propylthiouracil
- Radioactive iodine
- Thyroid replacement therapy
- Beta-blockers

### Mitral valve prolapse

- Beta-blockers

# 15

# How to Put Your Program Together

I hope you that have enjoyed my book and found it useful. I have shared with you a complete self-care program to prevent and relieve your symptoms of anxiety and stress. My program will both help to repattern your thoughts and emotions towards peace, relaxation and joy and also promote a healthier brain chemistry and nervous system. Your general health and well-being should also benefit greatly from this program.

I have shared many helpful and effective treatment options with you. Try the therapies that appeal to you. I recommend that you make them part of your daily routine so that you can receive the most benefit from them.

I usually recommend beginning any self-care program slowly so you can comfortably become accustomed to the lifestyle changes. People differ in their ability to adjust to major lifestyle changes. Though some of my patients like to eliminate their old, unhealthy habits as quickly as possible, other women find such rapid changes in their long-term habits to be too stressful. Find the pace that works for you.

**Enjoy the program.** I always tell my patients to regard their self-care program as an enjoyable adventure. The exercises and stress-reduction techniques should give you a sense of energy and well-being. The menus and food selections I have recommended in this book provide you with an opportunity to try delicious and healthful new recipes and meal plans.

**Try the treatment options that attract you the most**. You may find that certain exercise routines or stress reduction techniques feel better to you than others. If that is the case, practice the ones that bring the greatest sense of relief for your particular symptoms.

**Don't set up unrealistic or overly strict expectations for yourself.** You don't have to be perfect to get great results. Just follow the guidelines of the program as best you can and as your schedule permits.

**Remember that healing occurs in a stepwise progression.** It is never a straight line. Don't feel guilty if you miss a day of exercises. It is not a major issue if you forget to take your vitamins occasionally or don't have time to exercise on a particular day. Don't be discouraged if you can't follow the dietary recommendations on vacations, holidays, or because old food cravings become too strong. Everyone falls down at times. The successful person picks herself up and moves on. Just keep going back to your goals periodically and review the general guidelines that I've outlined for you.

**Be your own best feedback system.** Become sensitive to what your body needs and its messages. Your body will tell you when certain foods and/or emotional stress trigger menopause related symptoms. Remember that even moderate changes in your habits can relieve your symptoms.

**Periodically review the guidelines** outlined in this book and continue to adapt your lifestyle to the healthful suggestions that I have shared with you from my years of medical practice. Over time you will notice many beneficial changes.

## The Anxiety Workbook

Fill out the workbook section of this book. The questionnaires will help you determine which areas in your life have contributed the most to your anxiety and stress symptoms and need the most improvement. Then, by reviewing the workbook every month or two as you follow the self-help program, you will see the areas in which you are making the most progress, with both symptom relief and initiation of healthier lifestyle habits. The workbook can provide feedback in an organized and easy-to-use manner.

## Diet and Nutritional Supplements

I recommend that you make all nutritional changes gradually. It is important to eliminate foods that may be contributing to your anxiety symptoms and add foods that support your emotional and physical health. Many women find breakfast the easiest meal to change because it is simple and often eaten at home. To change your other meals and snacks, periodically review the lists of foods to eliminate and those to emphasize.

Each month, pick a few foods that you are willing to eliminate from your diet. In their place, try the foods that help prevent and relieve anxiety. The recipes and menus that I have shared with you should be very helpful. Use the meal plans as guidelines while you restructure your diet to suit your needs.

Vitamins, minerals, essential fatty acids, amino acids and herbal supplements will help complete your nutritional program and speed up the healing process. Most women find the nutritional supplement program to be a very important part of their anxiety relief program. The use of nutritional supplements can help greatly to promote a calm and relaxed mood.

## Stress Reduction and Breathing Exercises

The stress-reduction and breathing exercises can play an important role in supporting your emotional and physical healing process. These exercises have been designed to induce a state of peace, calm, and relaxation, as well as reinforce new ways of handling stress. When practiced on a regular basis, they also help build confidence and self-esteem. The visualization and affirmation exercises can help you create a blueprint in your mind for optimal emotional health and well-being; this enables your body and mind to work together in harmony.

Begin by trying the stress-reduction and breathing exercises that most appeal to you. Choose the combination that works best for you. Practice stress management on a regular basis and be aware of your habitual breathing patterns. Both these techniques will help you relax and release tensions. They will also help to repattern your nervous system and brain chemistry so that you are able to handle stress better and feel much more peaceful and calm on a consistent basis.

You do not need to spend enormous amounts of time on these exercises. Even 10 minutes out of your daily schedule can be helpful. You may find that the quietest times for you are early in the morning before you get out of bed, or late at night before going to sleep.

You might also choose to take a "breath break" or meditation break during the day. You can close the door to your office or go into your bedroom at home for 10 minutes to relax. Use the time to breathe deeply, do the visualizations, or meditate. You will be much calmer and more relaxed afterward.

## Physical Exercise

Women with anxiety symptoms should do moderate exercise on a regular basis, at least three to four times a week. Aerobic exercise can help to dispel anxiety and is deeply relaxing. It promotes healthy circulation and oxygenation and helps to promote healthy balance of the brain chemistry and nervous system. It is best to do your exercise routine in a slow, comfortable manner, so as not to intensify your symptoms. Frenetic exercise that is too fast-paced is unhealthy if you are already nervous and tense; it can actually stress and tire you out further. Pick a tempo that feels relaxing and comfortable.

If you are interested in doing the stretches and acupressure massage points described in this book, I recommend that you set aside fifteen minutes to half-hour each day for the first week or two of starting your self-help program. Try the exercises that appeal to you and offer correction for your specific set of symptoms. After an initial period of exploration, choose the ones that you enjoy the most and that seem to give you the most relief. Practice them on a regular basis so they can help prevent and reduce your symptoms.

## Conclusion

I want to inspire you that you have a tremendous ability to heal and that you can enjoy radiant health and well-being. By working with the very effective treatment programs contained in this book, you can create a much greater sense of peace, joy and relaxation in your life. You will also find that you begin to have a greatly improved ability to handle the day-to-day stresses of your life. Practicing healthy nutritional habits, exercising daily or every other day and doing the relaxation and stress-reduction techniques will provide you with great benefits.

By combining these beneficial principles of self-care, you can enjoy the same wonderful results that my patients have had in eliminating anxiety and panic episodes from their lives and enjoying each day in a much more peaceful, calm and relaxed manner. To your great health!

Love,

Dr. Susan

# About Susan Richards, M.D.

**Dr. Susan Richards** is one of the foremost authorities in the fields of family medicine and alternative medicine. Dr. Richards has successfully treated many thousands of patients emphasizing alternative health and integrative medicine in her clinical practice. Her mission is to provide her patients with safe and effective alternative therapies to greatly enhance their health and well-being.

A graduate of Northwestern University Feinberg School of Medicine, she has served on the clinical faculty of Stanford University School of Medicine and taught in their Division of Family and Community Medicine.

Her Facebook page, Dr. Susan's Healthy Living, has over one million followers. She is also an ordained minister and her ministry receives over a million prayer requests for healing each year.

# NOTES

# NOTES

## References

"Bioassay-guided fractionation of lemon balm (Melissa officinalis L.) using an in vitro measure of GABA transaminase activity" (http://www.ncbi.nlm.nih.gov/pubmed/19165747) . ://www.ncbi.nlm.nih.gov/pubmed/19165747. Retrieved 2010-03-08.

Aa *b* Li K, Xu E (June 2008). "The role and the mechanism of gamma-aminobutyric acid during central nervous system development". *Neurosci Bull* 24 (3): 195-200. doi:10.1007/s12264-008-0109- 3 (http://dx.doLorg/10.1007%2Fs12264-008-0109-3) . PMID 18500393 (http://www.ncbi.nlm.nih.gov/pubmed/18500393) .

A Barbin G, Pollard H, Gaiarsa JL, Ben-Ari Y (April 1993). "Involvement of GABAA receptors in the outgrowth of cultured hippocampal neurons". *Neurosci. Lett.* 152 (1-2): 150-154. doi:10.1016/0304-3940(93)90505-F (http://dx.doLorg/10.1016%2F0304-3940%2893%2990505-F) . PMID 8390627 (http://www.ncbi.nlmnith.gov/pubmed/8390627) .

A Ben-Ari Y (September 2002). "Excitatory actions of gaba during development: the nature of the nurture". *Nat. Rev. Neurosci.* 3 (9): 728-739. doi:10.1038/nm920 (http://dx.doLorg/10.1038%2Fnm920) . PMID 12209121 (http://www.ncbi.nlm.nih.gov/pubmed/12209121) .

A Ben-Ari Y, Gaiarsa JL, Tyzio R, Khazipov R (October 2007). "GABA: a pioneer transmitter that excites immature neurons and generates primitive oscillations". *Physiol. Rev.* 87 (4): 1215-1284. doi:10.1152/physrev.00017.2006 (http://dx.doi.org/10.1152%2Fphysrev.00017.2006) . PMID 17928584 (http://www.ncbi.nlmnih.gov/pubmed/17928584) .

A Boehm SL, Ponomarev I, Blednov YA, Harris RA (2006). "From gene to behavior and back again: new perspectives on GABAAreceptor subunit selectivity of alcohol actions". *Adv. Pharmacol.* 54 (8): 1581-1602. doi:10.1016/j.bcp.2004.07.023 (http://dx.doi.org/10.1016%2Fj.bcp.2004.07.023) . PMID 17175815 (http://www.ncbi.nlm.nih.gov/pubrned/17175815) .

A Ganguly K, Schinder AF, Wong ST, Poo M (May 2001). "GABA itself promotes the developmental switch of neuronal GABAergic responses from excitation to inhibition". *Cell* 105 (4): 521 532. doi:10.1016/50092-8674(01)00341-5 (http://dx.doLorg/10.1016%2FS0092-8674%2801%2900341-5) PMID 11371348 (http://www.ncbi.nlm.tiih.gov/pubmed/11371348) .

A Haydar TF, Wang F, Schwartz ML, Rakic P (August 2000). "Differential modulation of proliferation in the neocortical ventricular and subventricular zones" (http://www.jneurosci.org/cgi/pmidlookup?view=long&pmid=10908617) . *J. Neurosci.* 20 (15): 5764-74. PMID 10908617 (http://www.ncbi.nlmnih.gov/pubmed/10908617) . http://www.jneurosci.org/cgi/pmidlookup?view=long&pmid=10908617.

A Holmgren CD, Mukhtarov M, Malkov AE, Popova IY, Bregestovski P, Zilberter Y (February 2010). "Energy substrate availability as a determinant of neuronal resting potential, GABA signaling and spontaneous network activity in the neonatal cortex in vitro". *J. Neurochem.* 112 (4): 900-12. doi:10.1111/j.1471-4159.2009.06506.x (http://dx.doi.org/10.1111%2Fj.1471-4159.2009.06506.x) . PMID 19943846 (http://www.nebi.nlmnih.gov/pubmed/19943846) .

A Ivanov A, Mukhtarov M, Bregestovski P, Zilberter Y (2011). "Lactate Effectively Covers Energy Demands during Neuronal Network Activity in Neonatal Hippocampal Slices" (http://www.pubmedcentraLnih.gov/articlerenderfcgi?tool=pmcentrez&artid=3092068) . *Front Neuroenergetics* 3: 2. doi:10.3389/fnene.2011.00002 (http://dx.doLorg/10.3389%2Ffnene.2011.00002) . PMC 3092068 (http://www.pubmedcentral.gov/articlerender.fcgi?tool=pmcentrez&artic1=3092068) PMID 21602909 (http://www.ncbi.nlm.nih.gov/pubmed/21602909) . http://www.pubmedcentraLnih.gov/articlerender.fcgi?tool=pmc.entrez&artid=3092068.

A Jelitai M, Madarasz E (2005). "The role of GABA in the early neuronal development" (http://wwwiem.cas.cz/Data/files/pdf/neuroscience/2004/jelitai-2004.pdf) . *Int. Rev. Neurobiol.* 71: 27-62. doi:10.1016/S0074-7742(05)71002-3 (http://dx.doLorg/10.1016%2FS0074-7742%2805%2971002-3) . PMID 16512345 (http://www.ncbi.nlm.nih.gov/pubmec1/16512345) . http://wwwlemcas.cz_JData/files/pdf/neuroscience/2004/jelitai-2004.pdf.

A Khakhalin AS (May 2011). "Questioning the depolarizing effects of GABA during early brain development". *J Neurophysiol.* doi:10.1152/jn.00293.2011 (http://cLx.doLorg/10.1152%2Fjn.00293.2011) . PMID 21593390 (http://www.ncbi.nlm.nih.gov/pubmed/21593390) .

A LoTurco JJ, Owens DF, Heath MJ, Davis MB, Kriegstein AR (December 1995). "GABA and glutamate depolarize cortical progenitor cells and inhibit DNA synthesis". *Neuron* 15 (6): 1287-1298. doi:10.1016/0896-6273(95)90008-X (http://dx.doLorg/10.1016%2F0896-6273%2895%2990008-X) . PMID 8845153 (http://www.ncbi.nlm.nih.gov/pubmed/8845153) .

A Marie D, Liu QY, Marie I, Chaudry S, Chang YH, Smith SV, Sieghart W, Fritschy JM, Barker JL (April 2001). "GABA expression dominates neuronal lineage progression in the embryonic rat neocortex and facilitates neurite outgrowth via GABA(A) autoreceptor/Cl- channels" (http://www.jneurosci.org/cgi/pmidlookup?view=long&prnid=11264309) . *J. Neurosci.* 21(7): 2343-60. PMID 11264309 (http://www.ncbi.nlm.nih.gov/pubmed/11264309) . http://www.jneurosci.org/cgi/pmidlookup?view=long&pmid=11264309.

A Obrietan K, Gao XB, Van Den Pol AN (August 2002). "Excitatory actions of GABA increase BDNF expression via a MAPK-CREB-dependent mechanism--a positive feedback circuit in developing neurons" (http://jn.physiology.org/cgi/prnidlookup?view=long&pmid=12163549) . *J. Neurophysiol.* 88 (2): 1005-15. PMID 12163549 (http://www.ncbi.nlm.nih.gov/pubmed/12163549) http://jn.physiology.org/cgi/pmidlookup?view=long&pmid=12163549.

A Rheims S, Holmgren CD, Chazal G, Mulder J, Harkany T, Zilberter T, Zilberter Y (August 2009). "GABA action in immature neocortical neurons directly depends on the availability of ketone bodies". *J. Neurochem.* 110 (4): 1330-8. doi:10.1111/j.1471-4159.2009.06230.x (http://dx.doi.org/10.1111%2Fj.1471-4159.2(09.06230.x) . PMID 19558450 (http://www.ncbi.nlm.nih.gov/pubtned/19558450)

A Szabadics .1, Varga C, Molnar G, Oldh S, Barzo P,Tarnas G (January 2006). "Excitatory effect of GABAergic axo-axonic cells in cortical microcircuits". *Science* 311 (5758): 233-235. doi:10.1126/science.I121325 (http://dx.doLorg/10.1126%2Fscience.1121325) . PMID 16410524 (http://www.ncbi.nlm.nih.gov/pubmed/16410524) .

A Tyzio R, Allene C, Nardou R, Picardo MA, Yamamoto S, Sivakumaran S, Caiati MD, Rheims S, Minlebaev M, Milh M, Ferre P, Khazipov R, Romette JL, Lorquin J, Cossart R, Khalilov 1, Nehlig A, Cherubini E, Ben-Ari Y (January 2011). "Depolarizing actions of GABA in immature neurons depend neither on ketone bodies nor on pyruvate". *J. Neurosci.* 31 (1): 34-45. doi:10.1523/JNEUROSCI.3314-10.2011 (http://dx.doi.org/10.1523%2FJNEUROSCI.3314-10.2011) . PMID 21209187 (http://www.ncbi.nlm.nih.gov/pubmed/21209187) .

A Wang DD, Kriegstein AR, Ben-Ari Y (2008). "GABA Regulates Stem Cell Proliferation before Nervous System Formation" (http://www.pubmedcentral.nih.gov/articlerender.fcgi?tool=pmcentrez&artid=2566617) . *Epilepsy currents I American Epilepsy Society* 8 (5): 137-139. doi:10.1111/j.1535-7511.2008.00270.x (http://dx.doi.org/10.1111%2Fj.1535-7511.2008.00270.x)

A Watanabe M,114aemura K, Kanbara K,Tamayama T, Hayasaki H (2002). "GABA and GABA receptors in the central nervous system and other organs". *Int. Rev. Cytol..* International Review of Cytology 213: 1-47. doi:10.1016/S0074-7696(02)13011-7 (http://dx.doLorg/10.1016%2FS0074-7696%2802%2913011-7) . ISBN 978-0-12-364617-0. PMID 11837891 (http://www.ncbi.nlm.nih.gov/pubmed/11837891) .

A Xiang, Y.; Wang, S.; Liu, M.; Hirota, J.; Li, J.; Ju, W.; Fan, Y.; Kelly, M. et al. (2007). "A GABAergic system in airway epithelium is essential for mucus overproduction in asthma". *Nature medicine* 13 *(7):* 862-867. doi:10.1038/nm1604 (http://dx.doi.org/10.1038%2Fnm1604) . PMID 17589520 (http://www.ncbi.nlm.nih.gov/pubmed/17589520) .

Akhondzadeh S, Naghavi HR, Shayeganpour A, et al. Passionflower in the treatment of generalized anxiety: a pilot double-blind randomized controlled trial with oxazepam. J Clin Pharm Ther 2001;26:363-7.

Alan W. Bown and Barry J. Shelp; Department of Biological Sciences, Brock University, St. Catharines, Ontario, Canada L2S 3A1 (A.W.B.); and Department of Horticultural Science, University of *Guelph,* Guelph, Ontario, Canada NI G 2W1 (B.J.S.) (September 1997). "The Metabolism and Functions of y-Aminobutyric Acid" (http://www.ncbi.nlm.nih.gov/pmc/articles/PMC158453/pdf/1150001.pdf) http://www.ncbi.nlmnih.gov/pmc/articles/PMC158453/pdf/1150001.pdf. Retrieved 2011-10-20.

.Aoyagi N, Kimura R, Murata T. Studies on passiflora incarnata dry extract. I. Isolation of maltol and pharmacological action of maltol and ethyl maltol. Chem Pharm Bull 1974;22:1008-13.

Bell, Iris, Brief Communication. Vitamin B1, B2 and B6 augmentation of tricyclic antidepressant treatment in geriatric depression with cognitive dysfunction

Bella, R., Effect of acetyl-I-carnitine on geriatric patients suffering from dysthymic disorders, Int J Clin Pharmacol Res 1990;10:355-60

Benjamin, Jonathan, Double-Blind, Placebo-Controlled, Crossover Trial of Inositol Treatment for Panic Disorder, American Journal of Psychiatry, 1995; 152:1084-6

Bottiglieri, T., Homocysteine, folate, methylation and monoamine metabolism in depression, J Neurol Neurosurg Psychiatry 2000; 69:228-32

Bressa, G., S-adenosly-l-methionine (SAMe) as an antidepressant: meta-analysis of clinical studies, Acta Neurol Scand Suppl 1994;154:7 14

Chapouthier, G, Venault P., A pharmacological link between epilepsy and anxiety?
(http://www.sciencedirect.com/science?_ob=ArticleURL&_udi=B6TIK-442RN26-1&_user=10&_coverDat10%2F01%2F2001&_rdol&_fmt=high&_orig=gateway&_origin=gateway&_sort=d&_docanchor=&view=c&_searchStrId=1740815840&_rerunOrigin=scholar.googlE , Trends in Pharmacological Sciences, 2001, 22(10), 491-493))

Coppen, A., Enhancement of the antidepressant action of fluoxetine by folic acid: a randomized placebo controlled trial, J Affect Disord 2000; 60:121-30

Dhawan K, Kumar S, Sharma A. Anti-anxiety studies on extracts of Passiflora incarnata Linneaus. J Ethnopharmacol 2001;78:165-70.

Dhawan K, Kumar S, Sharma A. Anxiolytic activity of aerial and underground parts of Passiflora incarnata. Fitoterapia 2001;72:922-6.

Dimitrijevic N, Dzitoyeva S, Satta R, Imbesi M, Yildiz S, Manev H (2005). "Drosophila GABA8 receptors are involved in behavioral effects of gamma-hydroxybutyric acid (GHB)". Eur. J. Pharrnacol. 519 (3): 246-252. doi:10.1016/j.ejphar.2005.07.016 (http://dx.doi.org/10.1016%2Fj.ejphar.2005.07.016) . PMID 16129424 (http://www.ncbi.nlmnih.gov/pubmed/16129424) .

Erdri SL, Wolff JR (1990). "gamma-Aminobutyric acid outside the mammalian brain". J. Neurochem. 54 (2): 363-372. doi:10.1111/j.1471-4159.1990.tb01882.x (http://dx.doi.org/10.1111%2Fj.1471-4159.1990.tb01882.x) . PMID 2405103 (http://www.ncbi.nlm.nih.gov/pubmed/2405103) .

Fisher AA, Purcell P, Le Couteur DG. Toxicity of Passiflora incarnata L. J Toxicol Clin Toxicol2000;38:63-6. 10. Bourin M, Bougerol T, Guitton B, Broutin E. A combination of plant extracts in the treatment of outpatients with adjustment disorder with anxious mood: controlled study vs placebo. Fundam Clin Pharmacol 1997;11:127-32.

Foster AC, Kemp JA (February 2006). "Glutamate- and GABA-based CNS therapeutics". *Curr Opin Pharmacol* 6 (1): 7-17. doi:1 0.1016/j.coph.2005.11.005 (http://dx.doi.org/10.1016%2Fj.coph.2005.11.005) . PMID 16377242 (http://www.ncbi.nlm.nih.gov/pubmed/16377242)

Fugh-Berman, A., & Cott, J. (1999). Dietary Supplements and Natural Products as Psychotherapeutic Agents. Psychosornalip Medicine, 61, 712-728.

Gralla EJ, Stebbins RB, Coleman GL, Delahunt CS. Toxicity studies with ethyl maltol. Toxicol Appl Pharmacol 1969;15:604-13.

Hadjivassiiou, M., Headache and CNS white matter abnormalities associated with gluten sensitivity, Neurology 2001;56:385-8

Jape, U., Franke, I., Reinhold, D., & Gollnick, H. (1998). Sebotropic drug reaction resulting from kava-kava extract therapy: A new entity? Journal of the American.Academy of Dermatology, 38(1), 104-106.

Kuriyama K, Sze PY (January 1971). "Blood-brain barrier to H3-gamma-aminobutyric acid in normal and amino oxyacetic acid-treated animals". *Neuropharmacology 10* (1): 103-108. doi:10.1016/0028-3908(71)90013-X (http://dx.doi.org/10.1016%2F0028-3908%2871%2990013-X) PMID 5569303 (http://www.ncbi.nlm.nih.gov/pubmed/5569303) .

Lehmann, E., Klieser, E., Klimke, A., Krach, H., & Spatz, R. (1989). The Efficacy of Cavain in Patients Suffering from Anxiety. Ebannacepsychiatrv, 22, 258-262.

Levine, Joseph, Double-blind, Controlled Trial of Inositol Treatment of Depression, American Journal of Psychiatry, 1995; 152:792-4

Lichodziejewska, B, Clinical symptoms of mitral valve prolapse are related to hypomagnesemia and attenuated by magnesium supplementation, Am J Cardiol 1997;80:768-72

Maes, M. Lower serum zinc in major depression is a sensitive marker of treatment resistance and of the immune/inflammatory response in that illness, Biol Psychiatry 1997;42:349-58

.Mathews, J., Riley,Fejo, L., Munoz, E., Milna,. Gardner, I., Powers, J., Ganyguipa, E., & Gununuwawuy, B. (1998). Effects of the heavy usage of kava on physical health: summary of a pilot community.. The Mettical Journal of Australia, 148; 548-555.


McLoed, M.,Chromium treatment of depression, Int J. Neuropsychopharmacol 2000; 3:311-3

Mihic SJ, Ye Q, Wick MJ, Koltchine VV, Krasowski MD, Finn SE, Mascia MP, Valenzuela CF, Hanson KK, Greenblatt EP, Harris RA, Harrison NL (1997). "Sites of alcohol and volatile anaesthetic action on GABAA and glycine receptors". *Nature 389* (6649): 385-389. doi:10.1038/38738 (http://dx.doi.org/10.1038%2F38738) . PMID 9311780 (http://www.ncbi.nlm.nih.gov/pubmed/9311780) .

Miyasaka LS, Atallah AN, Soares BG. Passiflora for anxiety disorder. Cochrane Database Syst Rev 2007;(1):CD004518.

Mori A, Hasegawa K, Murasaki M, et al. Clinical evaluation of Passiflamin (passiflora extract) on neurosis - multicenter double blind study in comparison with mexazolam. Rinsho Hyoka (Clinical Evaluation) 1993;21:383-440.

Munte, T., Heinz, H., Matzke, M.; & Steitz, J. *(1993)*. Effects of Oxazepam and an Extract of Kava Roots (Piper methysticum) on. Event-Related Potentials in a Word Recognition Task. Pharmacoe ofincephalography, 27, 46-53.

Ngan A, Conduit R. A double-blind, placebo-controlled investigation of the effects of Passiflora incarnata (Passionflower) herbal tea on subjective sleep quality. Phytother Res 2011 Feb 3 [Epub ahead of print].

Pennix, B., Vitamin B12 deficiency and depression in physically disabled older women: epidemiologic evidence from the Women's Health and Aging Study, Am J Psychiatry 2000; 157:715-21

Petroff OA (December 2002). "GABA and glutamate in the human brain" (http://nro.sagepub.com/cgilpinidlookup?view=long&prnid=12467378) . *Neuroscientist* 8 (6): 562-573. doi:10.1177/1073858402238515 (http://dx.doi.org/10.1177%2F1073858402238515) . PMID 12467378 (http://www.ncbi.nlm.nih.gov/pubmed/12467378) http://nro.sagepub.corn/cgi/pmidlookup? view=long&prnid=12467378.

Pittler, M., & Ernst, E. (2000). Efficacy of Kava Extract for Treating Anxiety: SystematicReview and Meta-Analysis 20(1), 84,80.

Puri, B, Eicosopentaenoic acid in treatment-resistant depression associated with symptom remission, structural brain changes and reduced neuronal phospholipid turnover, Int J Clin Pract 2001;55:560-3

Roth, Robert J.; Cooper, Jack R.; Bloom, Floyd E. (2003). *The Biochemical Basis of Neuropharmacology.* Oxford fOxfordshiret Oxford University Press. pp. 416 pages. ISBN 0-19-514008-7.

Schelosky, L, Raffauf, C., Jendroska, K., & Poewe, W. (1995). Kava and dopamineantagonism. J Neural Neurtwarg esygliairy, 58(5); 63feW 640.

Schmidt, P., & Boehncke, W.H. (2000). Delayed-type hypersensitivity r coon to kava-kava extract. Contact Dermatitis, 42, 363-364.

Schousboe A, Waagepetersen HS (2007). "GABA: homeostatic and pharmacological aspects". *Prog. Brain Res..* Progress in Brain Research 160: 9-19. doi:10.1016/S0079-6123(06)60002-2 (http://th.doi.org/10.1016%2F50079-6123%2806%2960002-2) . ISBN 9780444521842. PMID 17499106 (http://www.ncbi.nlm.nih.gov/pubmed/17499106)

Seelig, M., Consequences of magnesium deficiency on the enhancement of stress reactions; preventive and therapeutic implications, J Am Coll Nutr 1994;13:429-46

Severus, W, omega-3 fatty acids, homocysteine and the increased risk of cardiovascular mortality in major depressive disorder, Hary Rev Psychiatry 2001; 9:280-93

Smidt, L Influence of thiamin supplementation on the health and general well-being of an elderly Irish population with marginal thiamin deficiency, J Gerontol 1991;46:M16-22

Spillmann, M., Tryptophan depletion in SSRI-recovered depressed outpatients, Psychopharmacology 2001;155:123-7

Wong, A., Smith, M., & Boon, H. (1998). Herbal Remedies in Psychiatric Practice. ArchGen Psychiatry, 55, 1033-1043.